SMART, STRONG AND SEXY AT 100?

SMART, STRONG AND SEXY AT 100?

New skin. New hair.
New YOU...

7 simple Steps to thrive at
100... and beyond.

David Kekich

What Others Have to Say about
Smart, Strong and Sexy at 100?

"As one who has devoted himself to radical life extension, and who has devoured nearly every book on the topic, I place *Smart, Strong and Sexy at 100?* at the top of my recommended reading list. David Kekich has managed to capture the essence of this complex topic and distill it down to a user friendly book. Whether you are a scientist or a high school student, whether you want to live forever or just an extra twenty healthy years, this book is a must read."

—Ray Kurzweil

Inventor, futurist, author of *"The Age of Spiritual Machines"* and
"The Singularity is Near"

"You can now live longer than you ever imagined. Allow my great trusted friend David to show you easily implementable ideas, techniques, technologies, lotions, potions and notions to grow younger and feel better than ever."

—Mark Victor Hansen

Co-author of the bestselling *Chicken Soup for the Soul* series

"Kekich is to be congratulated on this terrific book; informal but not superficial, informative but not over-technical, motivational but not preachy. As a specialist in the development of future regenerative medicine to defeat aging altogether, I want to see as many people as possible "make that cut" by making the most of what's already possible. Just how much that is, is still uncertain, and also varies greatly from person to person, but that doesn't invalidate the corpus of advice expertly compiled in this volume."

—Aubrey de Grey, Ph.D.

Biomedical gerontologist, Chief Science Officer, SENS Foundation

"Aging is the one health challenge we ALL have. Eventually we are confronted with the pain, limitations and weaknesses that seem inevitable, at least until now. Dave Kekich has compiled an easy to read manual that can help extend your healthy lifespan. The simple strategies he outlines will help to keep your body in good enough shape to benefit from the emerging technologies that should significantly extend the human lifespan in the next few decades."

"The book provides an excellent summary of contemporary life extension strategies and resources that you can plug into that will continue to keep you informed of the rapidly developing science of life extension. If improving the quality of your health and maintaining it for as long as possible is an interest of yours, then this book is a must read."

—Dr. Joseph Mercola

Founder of Mercola.com, the world's most visited natural health site

"This incredible book shows you how to live longer and live better, with more energy and health than you might have ever imagined."

—Brian Tracy
Author of *"The Way to Wealth"*

"Thousands of published scientific studies reveal how maturing humans can radically *reduce* disease risk and *reverse* premature aging. The dilemma is this wealth of knowledge is vast, and even dedicated health enthusiasts often overlook critically important components. *Smart, Strong and Sexy at 100?* overcomes this *information deficit* by compiling state-of-the-art technologies from the world's foremost validated sources."

"It is tragic that most of humanity wallows in a state of medical ignorance that results in the needless suffering of age-related disorders. Those fortunate enough to access *Smart, Strong and Sexy at 100?* will be pleasantly surprised to learn how relatively simple steps can inure enormous longevity benefits."

—William Faloon
Co-Founder, Life Extension Foundation

"You have written a very compelling and humane approach to a very confusing topic. Most physicians are not trained in anti-aging sciences, so it is up to the individual to decipher the protocols that will extend their lives. Your book provides a very good step-by-step guide to assisting in this journey. Congratulations David, you have made a valuable contribution."

—Dr. Gary Null
Author of over 27 health and healing books,
syndicated radio talk show host

"Many biologists concur that real life-extension technology—based on re-engineering the human genome—is predicted as coming sometime in the next couple of decades. But if you were to die too soon and you weren't here to take advantage of this new technology, who's to blame? That's why we all need a "Bridge Plan" to take us from today's science to that magical time in the future when death has been conquered, to ensure that we're still here when that day arrives. David Kekich's book is that Bridge Plan. Read it to make sure that you too are still with us."

—L. Stephen Coles, M.D., Ph.D.

Co-Founder, Los Angeles Gerontology Research Group

"David Kekich is one of the most dedicated leaders of the concept of 'Immortality', or as Kekich calls it, a 'Limitless Life Span'. In *Smart, Strong and Sexy at 100?* he has condensed the essence of scientific and personal data which we can use NOW to go on the express track for life extension.

Smart, Strong and Sexy at 100? provides easily available tools to maximize our inherent longevity and regeneration potential. We all possess these potentials to various degrees, all of which can be realized. Too many dismiss existing scientific data on life extension as not attainable in their lifetime, or ever. However we can, as Kekich says, capture and 'Ride the Wave of Medical Breakthroughs' toward a 'Limitless Life Span'. As Jerry Rubin stated in the revolutionary times of the 60's, 'Do it now!'

If you have any interest to live longer and better, then *Smart, Strong and Sexy at 100?* is a most necessary tool in your life extension tool kit."

—Karlis Ullis, MD

Medical Director, Sports Medicine & Anti-Aging Medical Group, Santa Monica, CA Author of: *"Age Right"*, *"Super T"*, and *"Hormone Revolution Weight-Loss Plan"*

In *Smart, Strong and Sexy at 100?* David Kekich has done what is for the most, 'the unthinkable'. He has posited the notion of extreme life extension – not in a trite, 'wouldn't it be nice way', but rather as a sincere and compelling agenda. The surprise is that because this book is serious about its ideas and conclusions, one quickly discovers that is becomes as much a book on morality as it is one on the science and disciplines of life extension. Read it and you will reconsider your life in a way you never did before.

—Patrick Gentempo, Jr., D.C.
CEO – Creating Wellness Alliance

Smart, Strong and Sexy at 100? is your navigational road map for a healthy and extended life span. Dave Kekich conveys dozens of simple steps you can take now to increase your life span, your health and prepare you for the scientific breakthroughs that lie ahead. A fabulous book that will make a major impact on your life.

—Joseph Sugarman,
Chairman BluBlocker Corporation and author of
"Advertising Secrets of the Written Word"

"Yes, you *can* reverse aging! This book not only tells you how - its author is living proof that it works.

—Ellen Wood
Speaker, Columnist and Award-winning Author of
"Think and Grow Young: Powerful Steps to Create a Life of Joy"

TABLE OF CONTENTS

ACKNOWLEDGEMENTS

There's nothing magical about writing this book—a book that could literally save your life. All it takes is surrounding oneself with experts in various fields, picking their brains, reading their books and articles and doing lots of research on the Internet. As Isaac Newton once said, "If I have seen further than others, it is by standing upon the shoulders of giants."

I have been very fortunate to have gotten to know many of these giants and treasure the pleasure of working with some of them. Most are not mentioned here because they contributed indirectly to this book, but they know who they are, and I hope they realize how much gratitude I have toward them for helping shape my life. Many work in disparate fields, which gave me the opportunity to help integrate their specialties into a formula designed to make 100 the new 50 within ten years… and another formula to keep you alive and healthy until we do cure aging.

I would like to acknowledge those who made a direct contribution to *Smart, Strong and Sexy at 100?* First, Ray Kurzweil, who may end up being one of the major contributors to extreme life extension, has identified a law, described in Chapter Two, that is the underlying reason full body and mind rejuvenation will happen before most people think.

I have been an active member of Life Extension Foundation for twenty-eight years. They are a world's leading resource of information on anti-aging products and services and have contributed mightily to *Smart, Strong and Sexy at 100?*

Dr. Aubrey de Grey may end up being singularly responsible for rescuing thousands, if not millions of lives through his engineering approach to repairing aging damage. He is also arguably the world's most influential radical life extension advocate. I have reported on some of his work in Chapter Four.

A treasured friend, Dr. Joseph Mercola, has managed to assemble some of the best natural health information on the planet and to deliver it to the general public. I thank him for much of the content in this book.

And thank you, Reason, for your tireless dedication to, and your analysis and commentary on, longevity technology breakthroughs. You helped make this book current and more interesting.

Dr. Michael Rose spent thirty-three years researching how to cure aging. He disclosed how to possibly live indefinitely by sharing his up-to-then confidential hypothesis on what I could do to accomplish that for myself within two years. I initiated Phase I in June of 2010. I am grateful for his potentially preserving my life as well as for getting his permission to share his conclusions with you in this book.

Robert Ringer has come up with incredible insights on analyzing the causes of chronic stress identified in Part II, and what you can do to chase it from your life. Dr. Stephen Cherniske has given fresh perspectives on optimal health habits and how to integrate them into your life. His information has also been a big influence on Part II.

I'd like to thank Shawn Phillips for his contributions to the section on exercise. And special thanks to Dr. Phillip Miller, Dr. Terry Grossman, Chris Crowley and Dr. Henry S. Lodge, Dr. Jason A. Deitch and Dr. Peter Hilgartner for their contributions to Part II.

I want to especially thank Greta Blackburn for her seed idea for the title of this book, for her wisdom and contributions and for her never-ending inspiration. Greta inspires with her actions—not with meaningless words.

Thanks to my friend and partner, Joe Sugarman, for all his sage advice on everything from layout to marketing. Joe helped make it possible for me to take enough time off to write this book while he worked overtime in my absence.

In memory of FM-2030, a futurist, author and lecturer, I have included some of his accurately predictive insights into extreme longevity and its positive implications on humanity.

A very special person and a new friend, Sean Stephenson, is the biggest man I ever met. Sean made important contributions to *Smart, Strong and Sexy at 100?* and I especially look forward to his benefiting from the ideas and sciences illustrated on these pages. Thanks to Joe Polish as well for introducing me to Sean among other contributions to my life.

My gratitude goes to Ron Hughes for the cover design. Ellen Wood has been instrumental in tediously editing every word, and John Lustyan has lent invaluable advice and more editing. And thanks to James Clement for his 1st edition edits and to Peter Passaro for providing me with some of the original content.

Finally, I'd like to express my gratitude to the thousands of thought leaders worldwide who relentlessly pursue their research day-in and day-out. These unsung heroes work tirelessly on their specialties, developing drugs, nutraceuticals, breakthroughs in stem-cell technologies, genomics, proteomics, anti-aging medicine, bioinformatics and other technologies, which are all contributing to your healthy longevity, even as you sleep.

PROLOGUE

It's been an exciting year, anticipating the cruise of your life—and finally, the big event has arrived. Here you are at sea on the world's most magnificent passenger ship.

The seven-course meal you savored was worthy of each of the five stars awarded the restaurant. Now, strolling the upper deck, hand in hand with the love of your life, champagne in the other, you pause only to steal a kiss under the starlit night.

Joyful music rising up from a deck below beckons you. A quick ride in the elevator ends with the doors opening to the most elegant ballroom afloat—adorned with rich, intricately carved woodwork, plush carpets, lit up by beautiful crystal chandeliers and alive with music and laughter.

The world is right. Locked in step, embracing your sexy partner, the two of you glide across the dance floor to your favorite song.

Suddenly, the spell is broken! Your senses are bombarded by the piercing sound and the shattering jolt of a crash... pain in your chest from being thrust to the floor... the playful conversation and melody has been replaced by an eerie silence, as you and the crowd stagger back to your feet and try to reconcile the moments before.

Questioning whispers become a hum of anxious speculation. Soon they erupt into cries of panic and mayhem, fueled by the fated doom coming to light.

True to human nature, there are people cajoling the band back into performing and partying on as if nothing happened. Those fearing the worst, scurry from the ballroom to the protective isolation of their staterooms. And others gain their composure, looking to assess the dynamics of the situation.

Soon it becomes apparent, the mighty ship and its passengers are in serious danger. The instinct to survive has people rushing for the refuge of lifeboats while some naively, diluting the severity of the threat, run to their staterooms to rescue their money, jewelry and other valuables.

Most of those, first concerned about their wealth, were dead wrong, and took it to their watery graves.

When the force of the impact was first felt, no one could've known that in just two and a half hours, the Titanic would break apart... and sinking out of control, would end its journey on the ocean floor.

During those precious one hundred and fifty minutes, some passengers remained in a state of panic, while those who slipped into denial, continued to drink, party, and enjoy the ride. The smaller percentage who kept their cool, planned rational action, followed instructions from the crew, and then initiated their actions. Which group do you think had the highest survival rate? Exactly. It was those who planned—and then initiated their plans.

As we now know, the passengers' hopes and aspirations for the journey of their lives, succumbed to the deadly and then unavoidable hands of fate.

Why Did This Happen?

That was the voyage from fortune to fate, for passengers, crew, investors and vessel on that shocking night of April 15, 1912. Not because they didn't have the benefit of breakthrough technologies, state-of-the-art equipment or lacked access to information about the risks in their path—but rather because, propelled by the journey itself and their sense of invulnerability, prudent preparations were overlooked or dismissed, and warning signs were ignored.

That course and those waters had been sailed for decades by ships of all shapes and sizes. The risk of ice flows was known and forewarned, and safe passage was within reach. Worse yet, they were ill-prepared for disaster, with only enough lifeboats for half the passengers. Denial? Overconfidence? Sloppiness? The Titanic's lack of preventative measures unnecessarily stole 1,517 lives from lovers, friends and relatives.

And they pressed on, full throttle... much like we do in our own lives. Focused on the demands and desires of our journey, we tend to overlook, minimize or ignore the warning signs along the way.

Worse still, when we do see them, we may feel invulnerable to them, push them aside for later or feel we have no substantial options. Like those passengers, our journey is nearing an end. Fortunately, we have more than two and a half hours—and far more opportunities to affect the outcome.

But how much time do we really have? Ten, twenty, thirty or more years? Hopefully, but we don't know for sure. What we do know is that we, unlike those unfortunate Titanic passengers, do NOT have a lifeboat to fight over. Sure, there are things to grab onto, to stay afloat a little longer. And like many of those who didn't go down with the ship and found something to cling to... it was temporary at best, usually prolonging the agony.

Keep Your Ship Afloat

The good news is, a "lifeboat" is being built for each and every one of us now.

Congratulations! By reading this book, you have chosen to survive, and the odds are you will not go down on aging's Titanic.

Like those at the helm of the Titanic, who in denial of the looming dangers, chose to go full speed ahead... society, including governments and corporations, are in the fog when it comes to aging and age-related diseases.

They party on, ignoring the reality of our pending demise. They dismiss the viability of building a lifeboat to cure aging. Instead, they tend to the sinking ship's maintenance, patching leaks here and there, bailing out water when it does get in, essentially just treating the symptoms.

Then when something critical goes wrong people panic. They pull out all stops to cure what should have been prevented. They never considered fixing aging in the first place... instead, passively clinging to yesterday's acceptance of the inevitability of aging and resting on arrogant pride at man's capacity to manufacture the next medicine.

All this works fine for the pharmaceutical and health care industries, because that mindset supports an extremely profitable business model. So together with big government, they create barriers to novel and even natural treatments that can cure or even prevent disease. This makes preventative medicine and lifestyle changes seem unwarranted and bothersome. So, most people march in step to the beat of big government and big pharma to a premature death.

Others cling to their wealth instead of investing a portion in their wellbeing and longevity—and the technologies that might prolong their active, healthy lives. Suffering, but financially comfortable, they die rich when they could have lived longer and become even wealthier.

Then there's an enlightened minority who seek the ultimate ROI, investing in their personal growth, and who invest in the type of technologies described in Part I of *Smart, Strong and Sexy at 100?*

This book shows you a clear and direct path to optimize your personal health... and how to prepare yourself for the impending technologies aimed at dramatically extending your youthful and energetic lifespan.

Maximum Life Foundation, a non-profit advocate for improving the quality and length of life, is spearheading the movement to make sure necessary research and development gets funded.

So who is the captain of your ship? If not you, you lose control to someone or something else. Whether it's government, big business or antiquated traditional ideas—that "someone or something else" rarely recognizes your individual needs and does not have your best interests at heart.

Are you going to let someone else steer you into an iceberg, or are you going to take control of your own destiny?

Obviously, no one would consciously choose to go down with the ship. Unfortunately, that decision is often made by default years before the ship sinks. As you know, insurance is not for sale when you need it.

So congratulations. You have now boarded the Longevity Express and will now be insured. Forget "sink or swim." It's time to jump that sinking ship. Consider reading this book as a step-by-step

shortcut and ongoing reference manual to your wellness and longevity. Reading it puts a safety net under you and fast tracks your
journey.

Read on to discover how this guide could unlock your door to
ever-expanding youth, growth and vitality.

INTRODUCTION

"Age without Aging"

W hy should we stop aging? It makes people sick.

How many times have you said something like, "I wish I were twenty-five again and know what I know now"? We can't take you back in time, but by the time you finish this book, you'll know exactly how longevity discoveries may be able to completely turn back your aging clock. And one day, you may look and feel like you're twenty-five again, but you'll keep what you have and know what you know now.

Only 100 years ago, the average lifespan in the U.S. was 47 years. Today it's nearly 80. Technology is advancing so rapidly, that you will be amazed at the progress we are making to extend your own energetic lifespan.

However, if we cure every disease, we still die. We tend to joke about aging, and then we endure it, until we get ravaged by it. Then it's not so funny.

Imagine the Ultimate Gift

What would you choose? A car, a home, a trip around the world?

How about extra decades? Twenty or more additional, happy, healthy, productive years. No cancer, no Alzheimer's... and a heart that keeps on beating! Twenty more years to spend with your family, to accomplish your goals and to enjoy life.

Since 1998, we've been hard at it, laying the groundwork for your ultimate gift. And a vibrant decade is only a start. What we are seeking—and expect to find—is not just a longer life for you, but a long, energetic and productive life; 80, 90, 100 and even more healthy years—with your heart beating strong. With you looking, feeling and acting like a person decades younger. We are constantly seeking out the best solutions, tips and ideas for longevity. We pursue research that can be useful to you now and in the future. Extensive studies are being conducted as you read this, in private labs and universities to understand what happens to your body as you age, and to find ways to circumvent or prevent the damage. We are acting now, because you don't have decades to wait.

Our job won't be finished until you put aging's decline behind you, once and for all. Maximum Life Foundation enlisted the world's best researchers to work year-round to let you enjoy endless holidays with the ones you love. Imagine the joy of watching the look on the faces of your great, great grandchildren when they open your perfect gifts. Imagine the warmness of sharing the holidays with five or more generations of your family.

If you're like me, do you too find yourself looking back from time-to-time? Do your thoughts ever go far back... to your best childhood memories? Nostalgic, sure, but isn't it a warm and pleasurable feeling? Now imagine never again being able to reflect on your past and never being able to plan for your future. What a horrible prospect, don't you think? Isn't it worth a little effort to extend this pleasure for as many years as possible?

You get what you expect, not what you want, so turn your imaginings into expectations. And imagine the best. Manifest a sound body by adopting healthy habits. Stay whole long enough, and we'll deliver the rest. We can do it, working together to build a long happy future for you, your friends and your family. There is strength in numbers, so help us grow our longevity community to help ensure your future.

An investment in your wellness now could pay off dramatically a decade from now... and maybe five decades or more from now. Remember, we're getting closer to rejuvenative technologies, and the longer you stay healthy, the better chance you have to be around when they can help you.

What about when life isn't so hot though? You could have serious physical, emotional, financial or other problems now. Dying may seem like a tempting alternative. But remember, many or most of those problems could be fixed within a few short years, especially with how fast progress accelerates today. Wouldn't a few years of low-quality life be a small price to pay for a soaring quality of life in the future? Refuse to let death be a permanent solution to a short-term problem.

To die now is like leaving just when the party starts.

Being Born Isn't a Crime, so why Are We Sentenced to Death for It?

So far, aging has proven deadlier than any poison, illness, infection, injury or weapon. You can avoid, recover from, or treat the effects of all the latter. But the 85% of us in developed countries who dodge death from those causes eventually die from aging. In other words, aging has killed 100% of everyone in the history of the world who were lucky enough to survive to "old age."

Life extension is not new. Just look at our past. From avoiding predators to developing antibiotics, we have always sought to extend our lives. Today's technologies simply expand this scope—live long and stay vibrant. This is a worthy plan for all of us.

Primitive man invented technologies to allow us to get beyond all our limitations. That trend accelerated throughout history. Extreme life extension is simply continuity between what happened then and what we're doing now.

Unless you're extremely fit and youthful now, there's no reason you can't look and function better every year for the next five years or more, or even longer, by adopting the seven simple steps presented in Part II. Even better, I see no reason why you can't continue this youthful trend for the following five to ten years by incorporating some of the products and technologies that are being developed, and will be developed during that time period.

And that's not the end by any means. Our researchers envision you recapturing your youth. They see you improving your looks, energy, strength, sexual prowess and overall wellness... leveling off, and ultimately being better than ever due to tomorrow's technologies that are being developed as you read this.

Is Radical Life Extension a Bad Idea?

You may know someone who might say, "I don't want to live for hundreds of years." That's totally understandable when you see how wretched old age can be without giant advances in rejuvenation therapy. Without those advances, I don't even know if I want to live to a hundred. But I do know I want to make that choice when I am ninety-nine, rather than having it gradually removed from me by declining health.

Most people don't readily accept the possibility of open-ended youthful lifespans in their future though. Many are even turned off by the prospect and consider death as a good thing. Why do you suppose that is?

Mainly, we have been conditioned from birth to accept death as natural, since until now, we have been powerless to do anything about it.

Old ideas die hard (pardon the pun), and the newer concepts expressed in this book are slowly obsolescing those old deathist ideas. But the general public is not comfortable with them yet, and many are apprehensive about the distant future. And their apprehensions are fueled by the entertainment industry.

Futuristic movies usually portray the future in a dark light. Central themes typically center around war; including class warfare, pestilence, evil mutants, death and all kinds of negative scenarios. The probable reality is things will be much improved in the future. Technology will deliver worldwide abundance, hopefully more peace and less envy, higher standards of living and ever-expanding possibilities.

Just take a look at historical trends. Standards of living, healthcare and overall wellbeing have greatly improved throughout history. There's every reason for them to continue and no logical reason for them to reverse.

But there's not much drama in portraying the future in a peaceful favorable light, and therefore little entertainment value in movies that portray peace and abundance. Also, the concept of open-ended life spans is hard for the public to relate to. Aging and death are familiar to them, and they don't relate to anyone trying to overcome or greatly postpone death.

So when media approach age reversal, they usually portray what they call "immortalists" as evil, greedy, ruthless, crazy or weird. To do otherwise, the movies might take people out of their comfort zones, and would risk losing at the box office.

Fortunately, younger generations have a fairly easy time accepting "radical" ideas such as open-ended growth. Older generations are much more rigid in their beliefs, and many may die prematurely because of them. One of the purposes of this book is to soften that rigidity.

How Long Can You Live?

You may be disappointed to hear we're not talking about living forever. If you're immune to the ravages of old age, that doesn't mean you would be immune to death. Accidents, violence, and other trauma could catch up to you. Being immune to aging simply means you no longer have a cap on the maximum time you can thrive. It means *you* could choose whether or not to grow and improve without limit, not your doctor or Father Time.

That's really what it's all about. Choice. If your doctor tells you that you have an infection that will grow progressively worse until it kills you, and then offers you an antibiotic that will wipe out the infection, I bet you'll take it—even if you don't want to live forever.

Yes, even if you don't much want to live forever, you still probably don't want to die today. Or tomorrow. Someday, perhaps, if that "someday" is undefined. But not today. And that's the point. A solution for aging puts the power to choose in your hands. Old age forces your hand. You don't get the choice to see your grandkids graduate from school, or to celebrate your fiftieth anniversary. The choice is made for you. And I don't see how that benefits you, me or anyone.

This is what it comes down to. Extending lifespans by defeating aging is not the point. At least it's not the main point for many of the researchers. The purpose is to alleviate the suffering that goes with getting decrepit, frail and dependent. Of course, this includes not just those who are suffering, but the suffering the loved ones endure who take care of them and who grieve for them when they die.

Extending lifespans is essentially a pleasant side benefit. It is something that will happen, because by controlling aging, aging-related diseases will mostly disappear. Then you will have the same ridiculously low probability you had when you were a young adult of dying peacefully in your sleep from an aging-related disease. You will live a lot longer. And I don't think you'll complain if you do.

Even though the original purpose is to alleviate suffering, the prospect of living open-endedly, with the strong supple body and keen mind of a young adult, excites me beyond description. When anyone asks me if I would rather avoid progressive deterioration—or live for a very long time, I say "both." How about you?

Longevity Express

I'm sure you're the kind of person who wants to avoid suffering and a premature death too. You're the type who appreciates great stamina, beauty and vitality, aren't you? Do you remember a time in your life when you felt you were on the top of the world, both physically and mentally? It sure would be fun to look and feel that way at a hundred, wouldn't it?

So consider this book as your ride on a revved up train to extreme longevity—an express that puts you on the fast track to that objective.

Has anyone ever taken the time to teach you A–Z, everything you need to know to add up to twenty quality years to your life? Boarding the Longevity Express shows you just that, depending on your current age, condition and health habits. You're going to learn things here that will supercharge your growth, longevity and outlook far more than anything you have seen before.

And as a bonus, it tells you how to thrive as long as you wish. This book could be critical to you, because *due to amazing future technologies, those extra years could be your bridge to an open-ended energetic future.*

You'll learn how and why you will see those breakthroughs, what some of them will be and how they will work.

So if you want to live long while looking and feeling better than ever, your answers are on the pages of *Smart, Strong and Sexy at 100?* If the prospect of limitless youth tantalizes you, you have just taken the first step to the best health you have ever experienced… for as long as you might want. The seven easy-to-follow steps in this book will transform your life forever.

Is there a catch? Sure. It's going to take some work, but not as much as you might think. There's no magic pill or quick fix to indefinite vitality, at least not yet. If any longevity fantasies are holding you back from taking action now, if you think some genie is going to pop out of a bottle and make you healthy or young, I've got some news for you. No one is coming. The information in *Smart, Strong and Sexy at 100?* is as close as you're going to get, and it's up to you whether or not you put it to work.

Now some of what you read might fly in the face of what you've been taught all your life. But these are different times, and everything you see here is backed by hard data and common sense.

So please keep an open mind. But if for some reason, you don't care about the future technologies, you'll still learn how to add 5–20 youthful years to your life.

How Old Are You Now?

Uh uh. Not so fast.

If your first impulse was to tell me how many years it has been since you were born, stop right there. There could be a huge difference between your chronological age and your biological age.

Let me explain.

Your chronological age measures how long you have been on this planet. Your biological age measures how you look, feel and perform—and is a gauge as to how long you will live. Recent studies have shown that the rate at which you age is only determined 25–35% by your genetics. The rest is up to you.

Thanks to recent knowledge, we are able to measure biological age objectively. It may not be precise yet, but it does give you a good measure of how effective your anti-aging program works for you—or how your habits may be accelerating your aging process.

For example, I have a young-looking fifty-seven-year-old friend. We compared notes on how we maintain our health, and we found our protocols and longevity plans were similar. He measured his biological age, and found out he was about thirty-five! I did the same and got similar results.

I'm seventy now (chronologically). Yet my blood pressure is better than it was when I was thirty-five and fit. (If you're not monitoring your blood pressure, you're ignoring a basic health tool.) My cholesterol profile is almost as good, and my body fat is about the same. I attribute that to my improved diet and supplements and continuing to exercise regularly. My skin elasticity, respiratory function and reaction time compare to someone in their late forties, and my immune profile, neurological scores and blood tests are equal to those of a fifty-year-old man's. Finally, an online test measured me at about fifty.

I say this not to brag but to show you how you can turn back your aging clock with the information you will find in this book. If my friend can do it, you can do it. If I can do it, so can you. We have essentially turned back our biological clocks by an astounding 15–20 years. That could mean we have each bought ourselves the opportunity to take advantage of over fifteen more years of nutritional, medical and longevity advances. That could be the difference between being part of the last generation to die from aging and being part of the first generation to live indefinitely along with those you love. Later in this book, you'll see why that fifteenth extra year could be as important as the previous fourteen combined.

You can do what we did too. You can. And if you cherish life, you will.

In fact, I have other friends who did the same. One was born sixty-four years ago, and he was dealt a bad set of genes that prematurely aged him and put him at risk of an early death. But through a well-balanced program like the one you will learn here, he was able to drop his current biological age to about forty-four. When he started, his biological age was probably at least ten years higher than his chronological age. Now it's twenty years less. So he netted around thirty years, ten years more than my other friend and me.

I have stories about other friends who do almost as well. These similar results are no coincidence. The Express will take you there too.

Once you see how you measure up, you can reverse your biological age dramatically. For example, let's say you are 50 and your tests show you are 52. That's not good. You have essentially short-ened your projected lifespan by two years and are expected to die at 79 instead of 81. However, let's say you start your Longevity Express seven simple step protocol now and retest in a year. The calendar will tell you that you are 51. But your tests might say you are 45. That means while you have experienced one more year of life, you are biologically seven years younger than you were a year prior. Now your projected lifespan could be 87, so you bought yourself an extra eight years during which new discoveries could be your difference between oblivion and youthfulness.

Most anti-aging physicians can quickly test you for your biologi-cal age. Ask for an H-scan. But courtesy of Dr. Stephen Cherniske, here are some free tests you can do at home:

Skin Elasticity: Lay your hand down on a desk or table, palm down. Pinch the skin at the back of your hand for five seconds. Let go and time how long it takes your skin to go back to its smooth appearance. If you're very young, it should snap back immediately. An average 45-year-olds' skin will take 3–5 seconds. At age 60, it takes about 10–15 seconds on average. By the time you are 70, it usually takes 35–60 seconds to crawl back. So if you are 60 and it takes 3–5 seconds, this test indicates your biological age is around 45.

If you want to increase your skin elasticity, follow the diet and antioxidant recommendations in this book.

Reaction time: Ask someone to hold an eighteen-inch ruler or yardstick vertically from the one-inch line. Place your thumb and forefinger about three inches apart at the eighteen inch line. Then ask your partner to let go without warning you. Then catch the ruler as fast as you can between your thumb and forefinger. Mark down the number on the ruler where you catch it. Do this three times, and average your score. A 20-year-old will average about twelve inches. That generally decreases progressively to about five inches by the time you are 65 or about 1 ¾ inches per decade. So if your score is seven and one-half inches, you test out at about age 50 for reaction time.

Games like ping pong, tennis and foosball can up your scores.

Static balance: Take off your shoes, and stand on a level uncar-peted surface with your feet together. Close your eyes and raise your right foot about six inches off the ground if you are right-handed, or on your left foot if you are left-handed. See how many seconds you can stand that way without opening your eyes or moving your supporting foot. Most 20-year-olds can do it easily for 30 seconds or more. By age 65, most people can only stand for 3–5 seconds. You lose about six seconds a decade, so if you score 12–14 seconds, you test at about 50 years of age.

Yoga, balance board training and exercise can improve your scores.

Vital lung capacity: Take three deep breaths, and hold the fourth without forcing it. Healthy 20-year-olds can hold it for two minutes easily. We lose about 15%, or 18 seconds per decade, so a 60-year-old will do well to hold it for 45 seconds. If you can hold your breath for 65 seconds, you test at about the 50-year-old level.

You can improve with exercise and deep breathing techniques.

Memory/Cognition: Ask a friend to write down three random seven-digit numbers without showing them to you. Ask him or her to say the first string of seven numbers twice. Now repeat the string backward. Do the same for the other two numbers, and average the results. A 30-year-old should score 100%. Most of the 50-year-olds will miss one digit out of seven. Most of the 60-year-olds will miss two, and 70-year-olds will miss three.

See the brain exercise section in Chapter Six to boost your memory skills.

So how did you test? Is your biological age younger than your chronological age? Great! Now you can do even better. Is it higher? Don't despair. Remember my friend who tested older but now tests twenty years younger? Starting now, you will do it too. If you're right on the mark, that also says you have lots of room for improvement. Who wants to be average? The average American isn't very healthy. Average means you get sick and die on schedule. Who wants that? If you test younger than your chronological age, congratulations! However, unless you're doing everything right, you can improve even more.

Going forward, when someone asks your age, why not tell them your biological age instead of chronological? From now on, I'm tempted to say something like "I was born in 1943, but I'm actually about fifty years old."

Maybe fifty years from now, you could say "I was born in 19__, but I'm actually about twenty-five years old."

What Will More Time Mean to You?

Let's come back to today. What will you do with 5–20 more years? How much more productive will you be? How much more quality time could you spend with your loved ones? I think you'll agree life extension is good, if your extra years are vibrant, strong, alert and youthful. And they will be.

But there's much more potential. There's potential to "rescue" the elderly. I believe inside nearly every old person is a kid waiting to break out. But that's not what the public perceives. They look at the elderly as disposable over-the-hill behind-the-times entities. So that's what most of us become.

I also believe people who act old have simply given up. They lost their hope. And by losing hope, they shorten their already limited remaining lifespans. We're hope junkies. You can't go forward without hope. You can't cure aging for example if you don't think it's curable. I love Thomas Carlyle's quote: "He who has health, has hope; he who has hope has everything."

It's tragic that many aging people lose hope, because as a group, the elderly are society's most valuable asset. "Old people" can be our most treasured resource. We generally acquire more experience, knowledge, wisdom and skills as we age. Rather than putting us "out to pasture" or in nursing homes, won't society be better off when we keep ourselves independent, youthful and productive? That way, we will use all the wisdom, experience and elders' extensive networks to solve the many problems facing us—and to mentor younger generations.

Imagine what you could accomplish if you had an extra thirty years and were armed with the knowledge you acquired in your first seventy years. Imagine the new perspective the elderly would have on life if they knew they were at the beginning of their lives rather than nearing the end.

The next ten to twenty years will see a revolution in medicine and the life sciences that will change the elderly forever. It can only be compared to the current explosion of computing power and communication. There is no lack of good biomedical science out there, but medical practitioners are typically slow to adopt new ideas.

This is for a good reason though. First and foremost, physicians strive to do no harm. But there is a fine line between being too conservative and being too ready to try a legal experimental drug or technique.

With the volumes of new information produced by scientists every day, it becomes a Herculean effort to keep up with even the narrowest of fields. The burden of staying informed on advances in a particular field will increasingly fall to those with the most self-interest in finding the correct information (i.e. the patients). Meanwhile, a support system is quickly developing. The medical specialty of "anti-aging medicine" is growing by leaps and bounds. The ranks of qualified practitioners are swelling, and the quality and quantity of longevity information is becoming more readily available through print media as well as the Internet.

Since you're motivated to improve the quality and quantity of your life, you can use www.MaxLifeSolution.com and www. ManhattanBeachProject.com to point you to some of the most cutting edge longevity information in the world.

This guide then is intended to inform you of the state of anti-aging medicine, and the current interventions that are possible to slow the aging process and alleviate some of the symptoms of its degenerative diseases.

Before we discuss tomorrow's extreme life extending technologies, you will learn how to use today's resources to maximize your health, longevity and wellbeing. We're going to start with:

Seven Steps to Set You Up for Extreme Longevity

They're simple:

1. Nutrition

2. Exercise

3. Nutritional Supplements

4. Anti-Aging Medicine

5. Lifestyle

6. Stress Management and

7. Attitude

This guide is intended to let you know that you do indeed have a great deal of control of your body's intelligence, maintenance and rejuvenation. Through these steps, you will greatly increase your chances of thriving well into the twenty-first century and possibly the twenty-second as biomedical science continues to advance at its current exponential pace.

Just when you reach the point in your life where you have the most to offer to your family and to the world, your energy, health and vitality usually drop like a stone. Just as things begin to fall into place—just as we come to terms with ourselves and gain the confidence to enjoy life—our bodies begin to fall apart. Why does a mind so full of experience and wisdom have to die simply because our aging bodies run out of steam?

The Express' seven steps will help make sure you continue, better than ever.

You may think you are doing just fine and don't need any more tips. As long as people feel okay, many get sucked into complacency and continue their bad habits. But under the surface, the consequences of bad habits insidiously accumulate until they erupt in the form of a heart attack, stroke or "sudden" onset diabetes or cancer. Then it may be too late for you. Too often, the first symptom of cardiovascular disease is a fatal heart attack. And did you know some cancer can grow for over fifteen years before you see symptoms?

Think about this: Your body is constantly whispering to you. When you abuse it, you get little signals such as slight chest pain, gradual weight gain, fatigue, pressure, elevated blood pressure, gastric distress and more. When you ignore the whispers, your body will eventually shout so loudly that you can't ignore it, if the shout doesn't kill you.

Consider the words in this book as whispers. Listening to them can avoid the shouts.

Your body is the foundation for your life, and you are the architect. You either limit your freedom from disease, or you build an unstoppable machine that churns out energy, vitality and joy, elevating your life and the lives of those around you—and increasing your opportunity for extreme life extension. Every day you stay fit and eat well, the gap grows between health and disease. You either grow or regress. Nothing stands still. Ignoring your health speeds up deterioration. The Express speeds up growth.

Would You Choose Beauty Over Longevity Though?

I had an interesting discussion with an old friend on the way home from a party. I asked her, if she had a choice between being guaranteed to live at least another thirty years or to be transformed to a twenty-one-year-old, but be limited to twenty more years of life, at which point she would die unless we were able to solve aging by then, which would she choose? She was fifty-three.

Which would you choose?

Here's what she said:

"I could have twenty youthful years, but I would die at age forty-one unless the aging code was cracked by then. On the other hand, I would be guaranteed at least an *extra* ten years of life if I chose to keep aging from now on, until science unlocks the key to age reversal, or until I die after thirty years, whichever comes first."

She chose the latter.

Look, she's as narcissistic as they come, and she won't mind me saying that. She hates aging and would love to be twenty-one again rather than staying on the path to eighty-three or older. But she chose at least thirty more years, even though she is already in her 50's.

She decided she'd rather see her looks fade and see her vitality wane in exchange for at least ten extra years of life extending research. She's one of those who know that because of the exponentially accelerating rate of growth, those extra ten years will see much more progress than the first twenty.

She reasoned that no matter how rich twenty years of youth would be, the chance she would take of age reversal not happening in those twenty years would be a sucker's bet.

Did I mention the billion dollar part?

She also threw a billion dollars into the pot. She said if she were made twenty-one biologically AND handed $1 billion, she would STILL choose her thirty guaranteed years over sudden youth. After all, she said, "In the big picture, twenty years is nothing. If science didn't deliver by then, I would have reached the end of my life, rather than the beginning." She added, "I'd rather start poor than die rich."

These mind games are fun to play sometimes. Of course, there was no billion dollar prize on the table, and we don't have the ability to take her back to twenty-one. But if we did, which might most people choose, short-term gratification or long-term satisfaction?

You'll find the answer in the next section.

By the way, studies have shown that children who delay gratification consistently scored higher on almost every measure of future success, including SAT scores, love lives and careers. A simple test such as seeing which ones deferred getting a marshmallow immediately or waiting and getting two later accurately predicted future performances of both groups.

Of course, delaying gratification is a habit that you can adopt at any age.

Stay Informed and Keep Tuned

This volume will continually expand as our knowledge of preventative medicine increases. Catching damage before it is done is vastly more productive than trying to piece back together a damaged system that we don't completely understand yet.

If you are one of those people who just can't get enough of all life has to offer and wants to squeeze every possible moment you can out of it, this guide will provide you with the tools to go out and get it.

More Life,

David A. Kekich,
CEO, Maximum Life Foundation

PART I

How and Why You Might Enjoy
Prime of Life without Limits

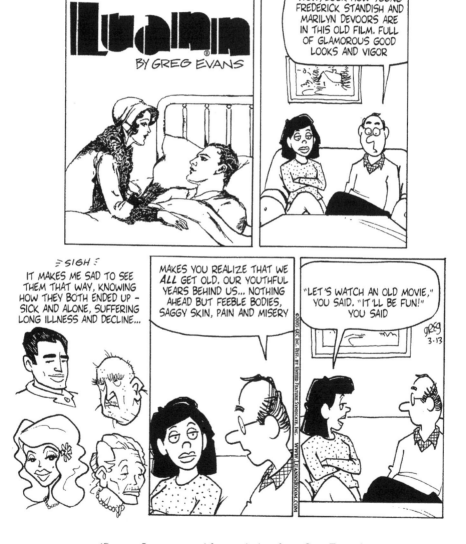

(Source: Luanne—with permission from Greg Evans)

CHAPTER 1. BACKGROUND

"Time is the fire in which we all burn."
— Dr. Soren, Ph.D. Physicist in Star Trek Generations

Almost sixteen years ago, on my fifty-fifth birthday, I went through the following exercise, which was developed by Mark Hamilton, to see how much time I had left to accomplish my plans. The exercise was meant to motivate me to use my time more productively and to help me finish those plans.

In order to illustrate how much time I had left to complete my plans, I drew a chart made up of 960 squares. Each square represented one month—for a total of 80 years. It looked something like this:

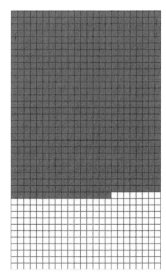

Note: Each row is
equivalent to two years

Oops!
I'm running out of squares →

You'll notice some of the squares are filled in. And some are empty. The filled-in squares represented the months I had already lived. Actuarial tables tell us men my age (fifty-five at the time) can expect to live to about 81 years of age. Then they die. The empty squares therefore represented the number of months I could expect to have left.

Well, to say the least, this wasn't very motivational. I noticed a serious problem. I already used up most of my squares. And the most healthy, vibrant and productive ones at that. And 189 of the best of the rest have flown by since.

According to actuarial tables, I now have about fourteen years of declining health and vitality left, without intervention. The frightening part is, fourteen years ago seems almost like yesterday. Is it the same for you?

So after some thought, I came up with a solution.

I needed to add more high quality squares. As I said, according to statisticians, I only have about fifteen deteriorating years left on this planet. But guess what? They don't know me, and they either don't know or are not factoring in the information in this book. Not only am I going to defy their predictions, but I plan to live a vibrant, youthful life long after they would have pronounced me dead.

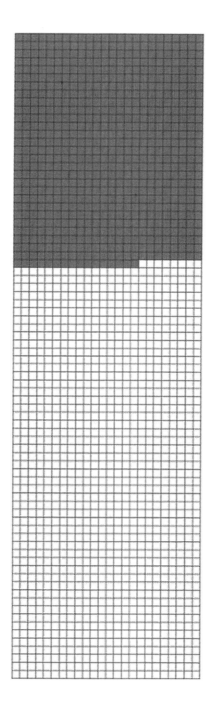

Some Personal History

Just what led up to the day I drew my squares? Let's go back in time for a moment to 1978.

Life takes funny turns.

Thirty-six years ago, I was a rising young entrepreneur who had founded what eventually became the largest master general life insurance agency in the country. I felt like I stood on top of the world. Besides the small fortune that was about to come my way, I enjoyed great physical conditioning. I was a long-distance-running, dedicated weight-training, vitamin-popping health fanatic. I was also an avid golfer with an all-star girlfriend, an oceanfront home and a new Mercedes convertible. I guess you could say I had it made.

Then a twist of fate dramatically changed my life.

On July 7, 1978, an obscure accident took place
in Manhattan Beach, California that could end up
being the most important event of your life.

That afternoon I was working out, without a care in the world, when something popped at the base of my neck. The next day, I found myself staring at a hospital room ceiling, paralyzed from my chest down from a freak spinal cord injury.

My injury eventually cost me everything—my business, my beachfront home, my girlfriend—a complete personal and financial wipeout. But most of all, it cost me my *attitude*! One minute, I was on top of the world—then suddenly, a hopeless paraplegic. Let me tell you, I wasn't much fun to be around for a long time after that. I was depressed, irritable, and even suicidal.

After a fifteen-month round-the-world odyssey looking for a cure, I "temporarily" moved back to my hometown, Johnstown, Pennsylvania—where I spent the next eighteen years supporting paralysis research.

What does that have to do with you? Just this:

*My unchosen path led me to a technological
strategy that could let you live well beyond
100 years of age, while being able
to dance like a teenager.*

I realized, "Sure, lots of hard research will let me walk again someday. But will I be young enough to fully recover and enjoy life like I did before?"

The hard answer was "No."

But I also discovered extending lifespans and even recovering some youth isn't much harder than curing paralysis. Many of the technologies overlap. Suddenly, walking took a back seat to a bigger and more important goal—dramatic life extension.

After all, if I could walk tomorrow, I'd still be faced with all the horrible side effects of aging—cancer, heart disease, Alzheimer's, fading looks, vision and hearing loss, diabetes, declining sexual function, loss of strength and energy and more.

If you're like me, you absolutely hate what aging does to you.

So I committed my life to conquering the diseases we all bundle under the umbrella of "old age." Why else did I do this? Because I studied life extension since I was in my twenties, I realized only about 250,000 Americans suffer from spinal cord injuries, while over 300 million are aging. I also realized I would be very old before I could ever walk again. I wasn't getting any more paralyzed—but I was aging.

So guided by some of the most renowned anti-aging experts in the world, I had a unique insight into how to extend or even save the lives of many of the 37 million people a year who die "prematurely" from aging-related causes. Then my long-term plan, walking, took a back seat to a bigger and more important plan—a dramatic increase in the length of time a person can live a youthful energized life.

I'm not a quack. And I'm not a promoter. I'm also not a scientist, physician, psychologist, nutritionist or even a personal trainer. I'm just an average guy who was forced into a position to network with the experts and integrate what I learned from them in order to survive. (My idea of survival is to live longer and more actively than most people think is possible.) I'm just reporting what is happening and am pointing out the direction in which we are headed.

And of course, I want to live long enough to cure my own paralysis. I want to run again. And I want to recapture the lost youth my injury took away from me.

Will I realize my dreams? I don't know. But I do know incidents like paralysis and suffering and the ravages of aging will be things of the past one of these days. And I do know we have an excellent chance to reap the benefits of those "miracles" in our lifetimes. I also believe the worst thing that will happen from our efforts is we'll add upgraded years to our lives.

Now let's go back to that day I drew my squares and conceptualized MaxLife.

Not only would adding more improved squares to people's lives be sensible and humanitarian—it would also give us a chance to enjoy long healthy futures. We may not be able to create more hours in a day or more days in a year, but there's a strong likelihood we can create more youthful years in *your* life!

Appearance over Wellness

A long life might not be the major motivator though. A few years ago, I had the insightful experience of speaking before an audience of health enthusiasts at a major health conference. I was featured as the longevity expert, and my speech was similar in content to the highlights in this book.

When I described some of the emerging life extending technologies and what they will deliver to the attendees, I captured their rapt attention. After all, if you traveled a long way to and paid for an expensive health conference, wouldn't you be interested in hearing about the newest technologies and how they could enhance your life and longevity? Sure you would, and so were they.

When I got to an adult stem cell technology that could regenerate or replace failing organs with pristine cells or tissue, the audience was fascinated with the possibilities of their extended and enhanced lives. I heard positive murmurs and saw nods of approval. But get this: when I mentioned the same technology could give them young skin and hair again, 1,200 people literally jumped out of their seats. The response was deafening. And I was shocked.

Here I was, informing a willing audience of the kind of health information they came to hear, but the strongest response I got, by a factor of at least ten, was when I told them they could *look* better.

This was a lesson instantly and well learned. It was also a lesson in frustration.

My life's passion is extended and enhanced *life*, not looks. And I want everyone to get it. After all, it could be a life or death proposition for them. Oh, sure, I want to look better too. I want young skin again, and I want the babes to check me out. We all want to be attractive. This was no secret. But when I got the most powerful response to better appearance from an audience of dedicated health advocates, it taught me something about human nature. That's why the title of this book is *Smart, Strong and Sexy at 100? New skin. New hair. New YOU... 7 simple steps to thrive at 100... and beyond* instead of something like *The 500 Year Lifespan*. Not only would most people not believe the latter, but they want to be sexy at any age.

As my friend Joe Polish says, "Sell them what they want (looks), and GIVE them what they need (wellness)."

The good news is, when you improve yourself on the inside, your outside reflects it. The quickest and most lasting path to better looks is improved wellness. Follow the seven steps described in Section Two, and you will look better than you have in years. Later, when the stem cell treatments are perfected, treat yourself to a skin makeover along with your new young heart.

Recapture Your Perspective

Remember how foreign or abstract death seemed to you when you were a child? Imagine how you would feel now if you knew you had fifty more youthful years ahead of you. How would you plan? What would you do?

Think about this for a moment: If I described the physical signs and eventual prognosis of aging to you, but you didn't know how old the person was that I was talking about, would you seriously consider the condition to be something nobody should address medically? Aging takes healthy, vigorous people and progressively leads them down the path to cancer, heart disease, diabetes, stroke, joint problems, overall weakness and immune dysfunction—and eventually kills them—without fail.

When we see these symptoms in children, we call it progeria. You'd be hard-pressed to find anyone suggesting we should just "let nature take its course" and let these children get sicker and sicker until they die.

Sometimes these symptoms start appearing in young adults—a sort of "late-onset progeria." This condition, Werner Syndrome, results in the initial appearance of rapid physical aging following puberty. Individuals with Werner syndrome commonly die in their forties or fifties.

Notice anything interesting about the Werner prognosis? Though the expected lifespan of an individual afflicted with Werner syndrome is actually comparable to the average lifespan of just a century ago, this condition today is considered something that an individual would want to fight against with all available medical resources.

We are finally moving from an era where nothing could be done to defeat aging into an era where advancing biotechnology will give us the tools to overcome it. All the old attitudes are no longer relevant.

We're so used to people dying from age-related causes that we accept it as a normal part of life. Aging kills slowly and pre-dictably, which is highly preferred by politicians and big pharma, who in many perverse ways, have a vested interest in the status quo. So we have become desensitized to this death. But let's look at it from a different angle and see if you think about it differently.

1. Robert Freitas points out 100,000 lives are lost every single day from aging related causes. They're scattered all over the world, so we hardly notice. But what if 400 jetliners fell out of the sky in a single day? We would be astonished,

outraged and sickened. Yet effectively, that's equivalent to 400 jetliner crashes.

2. If 400 planes crashed every day, wouldn't the world marshal all its powers to ensure aircraft safety, especially if we had no choice but to fly?

3. What if we could avoid—or at least postpone most aging-related deaths?

4. Then why isn't treating aging a #1 priority?

After all, if you or a loved one had a major medical condition such as cancer, heart disease or suffered a stroke, wouldn't you ask for the very best medical care?

If we had a treatment that could reverse Alzheimer's, Parkinson's, osteoporosis, arteriosclerosis or diabetes—who in their right mind would turn it down?

Now it is aging, the new frontier. Since it kills everyone who survives or dodges diseases, might not aging be considered a disease as well? MaxLife looks at it as a curable disease, in fact the mother of most diseases. And we're doing something about it.

One last thing: Many people ask, "When you succeed, are we going to be old, decrepit people living for a long, long time?" Or, "Gee, everybody has always died on schedule or sooner. It can't be any different for us. Aging is too complex to solve."

Many wonder if we will have an overpopulation challenge, while others have different concerns. Most are logical questions, and I have addressed them in Appendix B.

I had some of those same concerns when I got a strong interest in life extension, which goes back to before my injury.

Now, based on what I have learned from top thought leaders in the field, I know we will see the day when diseases are a thing of the past, or are instantly or readily curable, and almost always avoidable. There will be a day when serious injuries are going to be easy to repair, and where lifespans are going to be almost open-ended in active improving bodies. I intend for you to be alive and well when that day arrives.

Out of the Box

Much of what I have told you so far, and what I'm going to tell you about aging in the next chapter, flies in the face of conventional wisdom and may violate some of your most cherished beliefs.

I'm going to share with you *why* and *how* open-ended vibrant lifespans may be in your future. You'll also learn what you can do to increase your odds of staying alive and active until the miracles of technology will produce extreme life extending and rejuvenating modalities. And that doesn't mean keeping you older longer. We're not interested in extending your nursing home years. No, the plan is to keep you younger longer, maybe without limits.

To complete our plan of letting you look, function and feel like you did at twenty-five with all the wisdom and experience of your lifetime, you and I need to start with some basics.

Live Long Enough to Live as Long as You Want

Maximum Life Foundation has summarized today's knowledge, technology, products and services in this book to increase your chance of being alive and active when tomorrow's regenerating technologies are available. Consider this book to be a "Longevity Express." Use it as your personal survival manual, your bridge to tomorrow's life extending medical miracles. It gives you seven simple steps that you can take right now to add 5–20 vibrant years to your life. The exact number depends on your age, habits and current physical condition. These seven steps are synergistic. Any one alone can help you, but taken together, improvements become magnified. In other words, the whole is greater than the sum of its parts.

Smart, Strong and Sexy at 100? is probably different from any book you have ever read. If you're like me, you hate the physical damage aging does to you. Just when you're at the top of your game, your health and looks start going south on a one way trip to oblivion. However this Express hands you two keys.

The first is an understanding of why you don't necessarily have to follow the billions who declined, decayed and died from aging. The second key is how you can help ensure being among the first generation to achieve mankind's oldest dream instead of being part of the last generation "to die on time."

A decade one way or another could be the difference between death and youthful living again. Are you one of the people in that zone of uncertainty? Maybe! But you'll never know until it's too late. That's why the information you get here is so important.

Yes, open-ended youth and vitality could be in your future when you care enough to take charge of your wellness and longevity.

So are you ready to board the Express to an open-ended active lifespan?

Yes? Great! Then this book is for you.

No? Then ask yourself this question. Would you like to die within ten years? Ten years from now, if you are looking and feeling great, would you be willing to die the next day? How about twenty years from now? Thirty? Forty? Forget about living forever. As long as you are looking and feeling great, do you think you would want to die the next day—at any point in the future?

If not, you've chosen the right ride too. Our scientists say open-ended youthful lifespans are a near certainty, and possibly sooner than most think. But you may need to make a personal effort to help yourself to it.

Nearly every one of us hides under the sheets when it comes down to personally adopting life extending steps. If you ever need motivation, just visit a nursing home to see end-stage aging first hand. How could you possibly witness this and think you will never be in the same boat?

There are multiple ways to postpone age-related disease, yet the majority of the population ignores them. Sadly, that includes most of the nursing home patients who did nothing during their productive years to alter their course of pathological aging.

You are one of a lucky minority who are enlightened with the knowledge of how to delay the effects of aging. In spite of all the evidence that ever-improving youthful lifespans could lie at the core of your future, most people let the insidious antiquated attitudes toward the inevitability of premature death from aging override emerging life-giving reality. How many of these people do you know?

Here's the Reality

Human beings have longed for relief from the ravages of aging since recorded history, and most likely much earlier. For thousands of years, we raged and railed against death, but we were trained to prepare for it. Escape from aging has always been an unattainable dream, so we invented endless rationalizations for positive slants to aging and death. That's completely logical. If something is inevitable, painful and even deadly, then it's comforting to rationalize something good about it. Those rationalizations also give some purpose to life in the face of hopelessness.

However, for the first time in history, science is finally handing us the possibility to attain the "impossible dream."

We're now knocking on the door of extreme life extension. And many of us will obtain it. But many won't, simply because of deep-rooted beliefs from which we can't quite break free. These beliefs may be keeping many from doing what they need to do to take control of their growth and longevity. With today's knowledge and tools, you could keep yourself active and independent until emerging technologies turbocharge your lifespan.

In other words, many slowly but surely are unconsciously committing suicide. The stakes are so much higher now. Our unhealthy habits used to cost us lots of suffering and maybe 5–15 years of life. They could now cost you the brass ring—open-ended healthy youth.

We tend to delay or suppress thoughts of long-term consequences in exchange for instant gratification. We don't like to think about facing death. When we do, how many people do you know who rationalize it in one way or another and use its inevitability to justify "living for today?" What they don't take into account is, most people pay a price for poor lifestyles by going through a long agonizing decline prior to (a premature) death. Do you realize the average period of disability before dying is 3.5 years, and the average period of declined vigor is over 15 years?

The French fries you eat today seem harmless enough. But those bad health habits may cost you an endless summer of perpetual youth. With today's knowledge, we can expect to get old and *live*, not get old and *die*. With tomorrow's knowledge, there may be no limits to your growth and youthfulness.

Healthy living can be fun, too. And you still get short-term benefits. You will subtract years from your appearance and add more energy, strength and stamina as a bonus.

Don't forget, every extra year of health you gain can make a gigantic difference as the pace of medical development speeds up. Consider this. What if *one year* before a life extension breakthrough, an aging related disease catches up to you? Another statistic.

Maybe that breakthrough would have given you another ten robust years. Medical knowledge doubles approximately every three years now—and accelerates. So that extra year you added to your life better positions you to enjoy future breakthroughs. Now your chance for lots more active life suddenly jumps from zero percent to something infinitely greater!

Our Edge

Since most killer diseases are aging related, we're going after the root cause of these diseases, aging itself, in order to *avoid* or cure those diseases. While hundreds of billions of dollars are spent on cancer, heart disease and other research, and even more on treatment, we believe aging can be solved for a tiny fraction of that amount—if it's spent the right way.

And Maximum Life Foundation pinpointed and fast tracked that way.

Just How Long Can You Live?

If we can ultimately *reverse* the aging process through such promising interventions as described in this book, wouldn't this effectively mean immortality?

As we discussed, "No." We still have to account for accidents, catastrophes or other unknown causes of death. But many experts do believe we can eventually give new meaning to "natural" death and "old age" as we know it.

So we will leave your definition of "extreme life extension" up to you.

Robert Freitas points out that each one of us carries within us a unique and complex universe of knowledge, skills, wisdom, life experience and human relationships. Almost all this rich treasury of information is forever lost when you die. If the vast content of each person's life can be summarized in just one book, then every year, natural death robs us of fifty-two million books, worldwide. So each year, we allow a destruction of knowledge equivalent to three Libraries of Congress.

Consider. Natural death also destroys wealth on a grand scale, an average value of about $2 million dollars for each human life lost, or an economic loss of about $100 *trillion* dollars—every year. That's equal to two-thirds of the entire tangible wealth of the world.

Consider the social and economic costs of the death of a single individual with a significant mind. How do you calculate the costs of the loss of an Einstein or Bach? Even the loss of an aging father can't be replaced by his son.

Consider the fact that by aligning yourself with Maximum Life Foundation, you and your loved ones may get access to cutting edge life-saving technologies years before they are released to the general public.

Will You be Left Behind?

We are approaching a point in history where millions will be left behind. Others (hopefully you) will advance by leaps and bounds.

How about those who don't care? You love them, but they just don't latch on to your dreams for their healthy longevity. What do you do? Do you cajole them? Do you persistently try to "sell" them on the prospects of rejuvenation? Not unless you're a masochist.

Often, people who speak to their uninformed friends and loved ones of the prospects of extreme longevity get discouraged when their audience doesn't get it. Then they assume they will be alone after their friends and relatives have passed away. So they lose their enthusiasm and don't take the steps that will help ensure their own longevity.

Sure, you will lose some loved ones along the way. But many will eventually latch on to life extending practices on their own. They will join the ever-growing life extension community and will survive long enough to live in an open-ended future where aging has been repaired and avoided. Others, especially the younger generations, will outlive the era of death from aging and will enter the golden era of extended youth simply from the luck of the draw. Meanwhile, your lost enthusiasm could cost you your life.

Wouldn't it be sad and ironic then, that instead of leaving your friends and loved ones behind, you are the one left behind? Let's say you are the one who will miss all the future reunions, vacations, birthdays, holiday dinners and other occasions. Instead of you talking about the departed, imagine them talking about you—or worse—being forgotten over the decades. Imagine nearing the end of your life, regretting all your undone goals and aspirations, instead of looking forward to a lifetime of new accomplishments.

The next chapter makes it crystal clear why your prospects are bright.

CHAPTER 2. THE SINGLE CONCEPT THAT WILL CHANGE YOUR LIFE—AND THE WORLD

How can we consider extreme life extension now, especially in light of the fact that we haven't even been able to cure cancer after spending hundreds of billions over several decades?

Part of the reason? Supercomputers, like the kind now being used in bioinformatics. These computers can do experiments in *seconds* that used to take years. Consider health. As of just recently, we have the tools to reprogram biology. This is also at an early stage but is progressing through the same exponential growth of information technology, which we see in every aspect of biological progress.

During the past fifty years, biotechnology saw steady progress. Through trial and error, advances were linearly built upon previous breakthroughs. But it was slow, labor intensive and expensive. That's why, in spite of Nixon's war on cancer, we still haven't seen a cure after forty years. After all, biochemistry is extremely complex.

But it's a new world now. The biotech revolution of the 21st century will do for our lifespans what the computing revolution of the past fifty years did for human communications. Biotechnology and information technology are merging. We can turn genes off, add new genes to patients with new reliable forms of gene therapy, and we can turn on and off proteins and enzymes at critical stages of disease progression. We are gaining the means to model, simulate, and reprogram disease and aging processes as information processes and to reprogram our genes as easily as we reprogram our computers today.

Differences in gene expression between younger and older people are a well-documented fact. Restoration of youthful gene expression would enable cells, tissues and organs to grow younger as opposed to the degenerative downward spiral that now occurs.

Researchers will develop genetic engineering and stem cell therapies that will enable physicians to reverse aging, cure the diseases of aging and help us grow younger and healthier with advanced age. We are already learning how to do this. And equally good news is, only a relatively small number of master genes seem to be involved in controlling the aging process.

So far, researchers were able to increase simple lab animals' lifespans by ten times, entirely by reducing the expression of a few master genes. Others quadrupled a more complex organism's lifespan by effecting gene expression changes with simple selective breeding.

In ten years, these technologies will be dramatically more powerful than they are today, and it will be a very different world in terms of our ability to turn off disease and aging. It's also because several sciences and technologies are finally converging and working synergistically on the problems that face mankind. Specifically, information technology, biotechnology and nanotechnology.

For instance, medical researchers are now able to use supercomputers to speed up experiments that used to take years. The key? They're using a new technology known as "bioinformatics."

Bioinformatics is a computer-assisted data management discipline that assists in accumulating, analyzing and representing biological processes. Now they're adding computer simulations to accelerate anti-aging discoveries.

The major task of bioinformatics is utilizing the power of supercomputers to convert the complexity of the genetic codes of the human genome into useful information and knowledge that can be harnessed to understand the aging process and aging diseases.

The result? Faster and faster progress in the technologies that will give you more life.

It's not a surprise. In the modern era, our knowledge has been advancing by quantum leaps compared to most of human history.

For instance, scientific knowledge doubled from the year 1 AD to 1500 AD. But by 1967, it doubled five more times—and each time, faster than before.

Several experts estimate that today, medical knowledge doubles about every 30 months. That means we could acquire as much medical knowledge the next three years as we did from the beginning of recorded history! And the University of Iowa, Carver College of Medicine, projects that by 2020, it will double every 73 days!

Part of the reason? As I said, supercomputers, like the kind now being used in bioinformatics.

Here's another anti-aging advance: Research tools called "gene chips" can do tissue studies in *hours*—or even *minutes*—that used to take *years* of animal studies—or studies that couldn't be done at all. These gene chips are actually "laboratories on a chip."

World-Changing Concept

The following piece of information might impact your life more than anything you have ever experienced, seen or heard. If you don't learn anything else from this book, remember this. It is the rationale for light-speed progress in life extension discovery, and it may save you from a premature death.

It is the "Law of Accelerating Returns" as identified by Ray Kurzweil. That's the law that projects and illustrates the exponential rate of growth in technology as well as the ever decreasing cost of technology.

In the modern era, our knowledge has been advancing by quantum leaps compared to most of human history. As I said, medical knowledge doubles in much less than three years now.

So you can see the rate of change is accelerating. This means the past is not a reliable guide to the future. The twentieth century was not 100 years of progress at *today's* rate but, rather, was equivalent to about twenty years, because we've been speeding up to current rates of change. And, we made another twenty years of progress from the year 2000, equivalent to that of the entire twentieth century, to now, 2014. Then we'll do it again by 2021.

Because of this exponential growth, the twenty-first century is projected to equal *20,000* years of progress at today's rate of progress—1,000 times greater than what we witnessed in the twentieth century, which was by far the most amazing and progressive century in history.

One very misleading aspect about exponential growth is that it's slow at first, and then it's fast. So the future happens more slowly than people expect, and then it happens more quickly. Here's how exponential growth actually works:

Let's say you start with one grain of sand and double it every day. After five days, you'd have 32. Hardly noticeable! In five more days, you'd have 1,024. Well that's more, but not even a teaspoon full. In ten more days, you'd have over a million. Ten days after that you have 1.1 billion. And the next *day*, 2.2 billion. Five days later, you're up to your neck in 53 billion grains of sand. And so on. The first five days took you to 32. Now, in one day, you're choking on 53 billion *extra* grains. The next day an additional 106 billion!

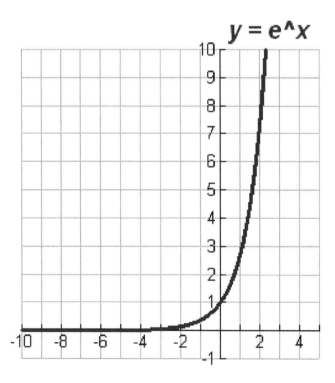

This is *exactly* what's happening today with knowledge and technology. You hardly notice the growth at first. Just like with cancer research so far. Then suddenly it seems to explode. Are you aware that the power of technology per dollar doubles every twelve months, and that the rate of growth is accelerating? This means our tools could be over 1,000 times more powerful in just ten years and a billion times more powerful in twenty-five years.

Now stop and let this sink in for a moment. Look back on the entire twentieth century and mentally calculate what 1,000 times more progress would equate to. Imagine what effect having tools a billion times more powerful could have on you and your wellbeing. This is an incredible, world-changing concept that will impact *you* more than anything else you have ever experienced. Almost all the old rules and restrictions are tossed out.

Human Genome Project

Here's a real life example—the Human Genome Project.

This project was controversial in 1990, just like extreme life extension is today. With our best scientists, Ph.D. students and our most advanced equipment, we managed to sequence (or roughly map) only 1/10,000 of the genome by 1989. Then, halfway through the fifteen-year project, 1% of the human genome was sequenced. Expert skeptics, and there were lots of them, were saying, "I told you this wasn't going to work. Here we are, seven and a half years into a fifteen-year project, and you've only finished 1%."

But if you double 1% seven times, you reach your goal of 100%, and that is exactly what happened. Contrary to many experts' expectations, the Human Genome Project was completed ahead of schedule and under budget. Just when it looked hopeless, progress seemed to explode for no apparent reason. But now you know why. And so did the key researchers. Where others saw little progress, where they saw only a 1% gain on the goal after 7½ years, the researchers knew they were half-way there.

They understood exponential growth. They know that going from mapping 1/10,000 of the genome to 1/100 was a 100-fold gain. They knew they just had to keep up that pace to get to 100%.

And they did. They shocked the world with what they knew was simple predictability.

Thanks to its predictable exponential power, only technology possesses the scale to address the major societal challenges—such as energy and the environment, disease and poverty. That was concluded by a panel organized by the National Science Foundation and the National Academy of Engineering.

Scientists now understand how biology works as a set of information processes. The approximate 20,000 genes in each of our cells are basically software programs, and we are making exponential gains in modeling and simulating the information processes that cracking the genome code has unlocked.

We also have new tools that allow us to actually reprogram our biology in the same way that we reprogram our computers. For example, when the fat insulin receptor gene was turned off in mice, they were able to eat all they wanted, yet they remained slim and got the health benefits of being slim. They didn't get heart disease or diabetes and lived 20% longer. There are now more than a thousand drugs in the pipeline to turn off the genes that promote obesity, heart disease, cancer and other diseases.

The important point is this: Now that we can model, simulate and reprogram biology just like we can a computer, it will be subject to the Law of Accelerating Returns, a doubling of capability in less than a year—over a thousand times more capable in ten, a billion times more capable in twenty-five.

Getting back to the Human Genome Project example, it took all the sequencing capacity in the world to complete. When the Project wrapped up in 2003, technology had improved to the point where 100 machines could sequence a human-sized genome in about three months. We're making progress faster, better and cheaper—and at a continually accelerating rate. Whereas progress used to proceed at a snail's pace, that's not the case anymore. We will see advances in the next ten years or so that would have taken over 200 years before.

Until recently, conventional wisdom dictated that if you live to age 85, you'll have a 50% chance of having Alzheimer's by then. And I used to believe that.

None of these projections takes into account the exponential rate of growth of medical and aging technologies. These projections completely ignore the emerging technologies and the impact they will have on turning the tide against dementia and other aging, medical and non-medical challenges facing mankind.

Here's something else to factor in: Our lives have become digital. Through the Internet, e-mail and mobile phones, human activities have become more accessible to quantitative analysis, turning our society into a huge research laboratory. Look what open source software has done to information technologies. Imagine what unpredicted impact the digital society will have on life extension research.

Finally, consider the fact that unlike research on nearly every disease where the work is being done by researchers who are NOT afflicted, most key aging researchers have a sense of urgency rarely seen in other labs. They are driven by their own keen awareness of what aging is doing to them and their families. Their lives are on the line.

Now, medical research moves 10,000 times as fast as it did twenty years ago. Progress is approaching the speed of light! And MaxLife positions you directly in the path of this major trend.

This is why life extending and cancer and heart disease technologies, which seemed to be advancing agonizingly slow, are about to go into hyperdrive.

Read That Last Section Again

So now you can answer all the so called "experts" who proclaim "extreme life extension is not possible, at least in the foreseeable future." You have the advantage of understanding the Law of Accelerating Returns, an almost unknown law that will catch the world off guard and improve it in ways most people could never imagine.

If you're skeptical, keep in mind that Kurzweil has a twenty-seven-year track record as a futurist. Many of the predictions in his 1990 bestseller, *The Age of Intelligent Machines*, such as the rise of the Internet, have tracked very accurately. Then there are his numerous awards, including nineteen honorary Ph.D.s and the 1999 National Medal of Technology, which Kurzweil accepted from President Bill Clinton. *Forbes* has called him "the ultimate thinking machine," and *Inc.* has said he is "Edison's rightful heir." And in 2011, TIME Magazine's Poll named him the "30th most influential person in the world."

The Law of Accelerating Returns is one of the reasons why there will be dramatic interventions in the aging process in the near future and why you have a chance to benefit from them. Things are going to happen so much faster and so much more dramatically in biology that it is going to benefit you in ways you couldn't imagine. But you will only benefit from those if you are still alive. So hang on for a good ride, and take care of yourself now.

It Gets Cheaper, Too

Here are examples of how powerful the Law of Accelerating Returns' 50% annual deflationary factor is.

In 1965, MIT, one of the world's most technologically advanced universities, had one computer. Housed in its own building, it cost $11 million (in today's dollars) and was shared by all students and faculty. Four decades later, the computer in your cellphone is a million times smaller, a million times less expensive and thousands of times more powerful. That's over a billion-fold increase in the amount of computation you can buy per dollar.

Yet as powerful as information technology is today, we will make another billion-fold increase in capability (for the same cost) over the next twenty-five years.

The Human Genome Project was completed in April 2003 for roughly $3 billion. Then in May 2007, Dr. James Watson's genome was sequenced for about $1 million or 3,000 times cheaper! In late 2007, two companies offered to sequence anyone's genome for $350,000. By late March, 2008, Applied Biosystems did one for $60,000 in six weeks, excluding labor, and recently announced their new system will enable scientists to sequence a human genome for approximately $10,000.

Then out of nowhere, a company called Complete Genomics announced the industry shattering claim of $5,000 for sequencing a whole human genome in 2009. This year, Complete Genomics is aiming to sequence a whopping one million human genomes! Here is a company that nobody had even heard of until it came out of stealth mode in October 2008, and it may dominate this multi-billion dollar industry.

Fast forward to January 14, 2014. Illumina, Inc. made a media splash announcement… reaching the major biotech milestone of the first $1,000 genome.

Recently, when the longtime goal of a $1,000 genome was not quite here, a Harvard University physicist promised an even cheaper price—the ability to sequence a human genome for just $30. David Weitz and his team are adapting microfluidics technology that uses tiny droplets, a strategy developed in his lab, to DNA sequencing. While the researchers have not yet sequenced DNA, they have successfully demonstrated parts of the process and formed a startup, GnuBio, to commercialize the technology. Weitz presented the findings at the Consumer Genomics Conference in Boston.

> "The twin incentives for engineering greater human longevity: on the one hand, we have the stick of disease, degeneration, and suffering. On the other hand we have the carrot of a life that in all other aspects generally keeps getting better. Being older brings with it wisdom, knowledge, experience, and perhaps most importantly independence—the ability to be your own person and forge your own path. Youth is wasted on the young, as they say, so why not work at making youth available to everyone? It's the horror of the human condition that just as we get to the point of being practiced and elegant, the rug is pulled out from under us. But engineered healthy longevity is a very possible, plausible goal for this present age of biotechnology. Like all good things, it requires work to realize: the longer we hang around not working on it, the longer it'll take to arrive."

How many more companies do you suppose are silently working behind the scenes to turbocharge your lifespan? Keep yourself ticking long enough to find out.

Do you realize the implications to your personal growth and longevity? Researchers could zero in on the mutations that cause Alzheimer's, cancer, aging and more. Your doctors will be able to predict the infirmities that are poised to trip you up and head them off before they strike you down. Drug and biotech companies will be better-equipped to develop more precise and more powerful drugs to prevent or cure your diseases.

My hot button is identifying the genes that contribute most to longevity and aging and developing ways to express the longevity genes to make you live longer and better, and to suppress the genes that prematurely age you. There's even more potential, but you get the idea.

Another reason cost will plummet is reflected by a recent Daniel Grushkin article in *Newsweek*. He reports that Tom Knight, a tech-guru-cum-biotech-patron, says the Biotech Age will do to the physical world what the Information Age has done to data. His thesis is rooted in the cell, which he considers the most perfect manufacturing platform ever made.

"I think there's a good chance we can transition from a world where manufacturing is capital-intensive to one where the cost of manufacturing is on the same par with the cost of replicating information," Knight says. In other words, the majority of manufacturing capital won't be spent on raw materials and machinery. Rapidly reproducing cells can take care of that. In a sense, the cells will behave both as the factory and the product.

Looking Backwards

Now that you see how quickly we are advancing, let's peek into the past by *stepping back in time for a moment.*

In 2006, I visited the famous Mission San Juan Capistrano in Southern California. It was an eye-opening experience for me.

It was founded in 1776 and completed in 1806, almost exactly 200 years before my visit. Two hundred years is a very short time in the grand scheme of things—almost recent history. The mission is like a time capsule, completely surrounded by a modern upscale town. Not only is the compound 200 years old, but it's basically a museum, a snapshot of time in sharp contrast to the twenty-first century life on the other side of its walls.

Because of my acute sensitivity to today's rapid rate of progress (after all, that's our master key to super longevity) the impact of how people lived in those days had special meaning to me.

Life was crude then. And tough. And short. Most people worked morning to night just to survive. And that didn't work very well either. They lived hard and died young. Their average lifespan was about thirty-seven years.

From the time the mission was founded until it was completed, thirty years, life didn't change much. People had basically the same tools, lifestyles and experiences that their parents and grandparents had. They had virtually nothing compared with what we take for granted today. They had no cell phones, in fact, no phones at all. No Internet, computers, TVs, radios or movies. If they wanted to go somewhere, they either walked or, if they were lucky, rode a horse or in a wagon. They didn't even dream of electricity, gas, central heating or air conditioning. They couldn't imagine hot and cold running water—or even toilets.

While I was contemplating this, I had a cell phone in my pocket that could instantly connect me to almost anyone, anywhere in the world and to almost every bit of recorded information on the planet. And this technology, all of it, sprung into existence in less than the thirty years it took to build the mission.

In 1976, there was no Internet, and there were no cell phones. As for PCs? Forget it. Microsoft was only founded in 1975, and a year later, Apple Computer.

I was struck by the contrast between almost zero changes from 1776–1806 and the revolutionary changes from 1976–2006.

I trust this illustration of how things are speeding up helps you appreciate the concept of exponential growth, how it will keep accelerating life extension technologies and the effect it could have on you and your health and longevity. I urge you to do everything in your power to outlive death from aging. Your payoff will be *huge*. And the best news is you can get maximum benefits in minimum time. By following the seven steps in this book, the amount of time and effort you need to commit is ridiculously small compared to your rewards.

So here's a simple Longevity Express formula for you to internalize:

Minimum time invested now = Maximum extra time later

CHAPTER 3. WHAT IS AGING, AND WHAT CAN YOU DO ABOUT IT NOW?

Before discussing the possible ways of slowing the aging process, we at Maximum Life Foundation first want to address what the aging process actually is.

Aging is an exponential increase of the probability of weakness, disease and death with age.

In humans, it begins at approximately twenty-five years of age in women and twenty-eight years of age in men. Some think it begins much earlier in life. There has been a long debate in the annals of medicine over whether aging is a disease or a natural process. Aging can be construed as natural only in the respect that it happens to all humans. But what happens is a collection of one or more degenerative processes that eventually lead to death. Aging is definitely complex.

Aging's complexity can be illustrated with your genome. For example, there are at least eight dissimilar genetic pathways involved in longevity; inflammation, oxidative stress and six others.

Most agree aging is the accumulation of damage at the cellular level. Some say we are genetically programmed to age. In that case, DNA errors damage the fragile molecular machinery of our cells. The buildup of genetic errors ends up causing the symptoms that we call "diseases"... which usually kill us.

The top four causes of death (1. heart disease; 2. cancer; 3. stroke; and 4. arterial blockages) are directly linked to the process of aging. Of the top fifteen causes of death, only four are not related to aging (accidents, HIV, suicide, and murder). Collectively then, the group of degenerative diseases we term "aging" are directly responsible for the deaths of roughly 85% of all the deaths in the United States (see figure on next page).

We have already cured what used to kill most humans. The three leading causes of death in 1900 were pneumonia, tuberculosis and diarrhea.

Starting in 1840, the British government provided smallpox vaccinations free of charge. Yet more than 500 million people died of smallpox worldwide before it was finally eradicated in 1980—140 years later!

I wonder if in the next fifty years or so, someone will write that we had the knowledge at our disposal to cure aging sooner, but an entire generation was lost because not enough resources were allocated to tie the scientific pieces together.

Leading Causes of Death in the U.S. (2002)

Ranking	Disease Category	Number of deaths
	All causes	2,443,387
1	Diseases of heart	696,947
2	Malignant neoplasms	557,271
3	Cerebrovascular diseases	162,672
4	Chronic lower respiratory diseases	124,816
5	Unintentional injuries	106,742
6	Diabetes mellitus	73,249
7	Influenza and pneumonia	65,681
8	Alzheimer's disease	58,866
9	Nephritis, nephrotic syndrome, and nephrosis	40,974
10	Septicemia	33,865

SOURCE: National Vital Statistics Reports, Deaths: Leading Causes for 2002, October 2004

Are these deaths preventable, and should we stop them if we can? Our opinion is an emphatic *"yes!"* on both counts.

Take Alzheimer's, Parkinson's, osteoporosis, atherosclerosis and diabetes. The underlying processes of aging are what tie these diseases together.

Can we cure each of these diseases then? Each of these processes has a definable cause. All of the causes are not yet known, but many are. For example, for a few years now, scientists have had a very good understanding of the basic mechanisms behind cancer.

Cancer is caused by physical, chemical, or viral damage to a cell's DNA, which in turn short-circuits that cell's ability to control its own growth and act as part of an organism. It becomes a group of rogue cells reproducing as fast as they can, stealing the resources of the rest of the organism of which they are a part.

If you ask any physician if most cancer is preventable, the answer should be a resounding "yes." The National Cancer Institute estimates 80% of all cancers are preventable. Of course, genetics can contribute to the likelihood of having cancer, but it is primarily the result of our environment imposing constant damage to your body. By controlling what food you eat, the water you drink, the air you breathe, the radiation you experience and what chemicals you expose yourself to, you can drastically reduce the amount of damage you accumulate in your DNA over the course of your life.

The same rings true with cardiovascular disease. It's actually quite simple to avoid. Let's start with balancing your blood lipid levels.

The most effective way to optimize your cholesterol profile and prevent heart disease is with diet and exercise. Did you know 75 percent of your cholesterol is produced by your liver, which is influenced by your insulin levels?

Therefore, if you optimize your insulin level, you will automatically optimize your cholesterol and reduce your risk of both diabetes and heart disease. The underlying cause is insulin resistance caused by eating too many sugars, grains and especially fructose.

The best ways to safely regulate your cholesterol and reduce your risk of our #1 killer, heart disease, include:

- Gradually reduce, until you eliminate grains and fructose from your diet.

- Get plenty of high quality, animal-based omega-3 fats, and reduce your consumption of damaged omega-6 fats (trans fats, vegetable oils).

- Include heart-healthy foods in your diet, such as olive oil, coconut and coconut oil, organic eggs, avocados, raw nuts and seeds and organic grass-fed meats.

- Optimize your vitamin D levels.

- Exercise six to seven days a week.

- Don't smoke, and moderate you alcohol consumption.

- Get plenty of good quality sleep.

More on all these life-enhancers in Part II.

Rocket Science?

Many of the techniques we discuss in this book may seem like common sense at first glance. You know you should be eating a healthier diet, exercising, not smoking and not drinking as much. Why, though?

The human body is a wonderfully complex machine. This machine is designed to repair itself in the event of damage. For the most part, it does a terrific job. But for reasons we don't completely understand yet, many of these repair systems break down as we age, and we suffer damage.

Mutations to our DNA occur when cells divide and mistakes accumulate. In turn cells become dysfunctional, cancerous or outright die. Other cells, including stem cells, can take the place of many errant cells, but these are limited in number and also eventually age and/or are depleted.

Many inadequate mechanisms probably include:

➤ Drift in control of how your genes are expressed, or turned on or off, and maintenance of your chromosome structure. This includes drift in chemical modifications to your DNA (your genetic instructions, the hereditary material in your cells).

➤ Accumulation of damaged proteins, lipofuscin ("age pigment") and other waste products in our cells that are not excreted efficiently from the cells or the body.

➤ Oxidative damage including damage to cell membranes, mitochondria (your cell's power plants), DNA, enzymes, etc.

➤ Damage to proteins and other long-lived molecules.

➤ Damage to DNA and breaks both in the mitochondrial and nuclear genomes.

It is also clear that the more you abuse your body by insulting it with toxic substances, the more likely one of your repair systems will undergo an early breakdown.

One of the most prevalent types of damage to your body is caused by a type of molecule referred to as a "free radical" or a "reactive oxygen species" (ROS) that causes oxidative damage, or oxidative stress. These are molecules that are produced on a regular basis in the energy generation part of your cells—the mitochondria. These tiny power plants are the final step in converting the food you eat into a useable form of energy for your cells. During the process, oxygen is used to produce highly reactive molecules that are normally well contained in your mitochondria, which has multiple antioxidant systems for cleaning them up and making them less reactive.

As we age, and in times of stress or extreme exertion, these systems cannot always keep up with the amount of ROSs being produced. These molecules, free of the mitochondria, can do tremendous amounts of damage to nearby tissues. In addition, the cells of your immune system also release ROSs for the purpose of destroying invaders. This is part of the reason why inflammation can sometimes do more harm than it does good because it can destroy your own tissue along with the invaders.

Basically, inflammation is a defensive reaction to infections, toxins or injury. The swellings around cuts, sprains or mosquito bites are common examples. It also happens insidiously inside your body.

Reducing this body-wide inflammation can slash your chances of heart disease and cancer *in half* and may be the key to Alzheimer's, arthritis and diabetes. Inflammation lies at the core of most chronic age-related diseases. It is also associated with high levels of acidity.

One of the molecules most severely affected by ROSs is deoxyribonucleic acid (DNA). DNA is the material that makes up your genes, or the very storehouse of the information that makes you, *you*. When DNA reacts with an ROS it can change the shape of or mutate part of the DNA and possibly cause certain genes to be turned off, turned on, or destroyed inappropriately. If these disruptions affect critical genes, many times the result is a cancerous cell.

Crosslinking

Another type of damage caused by ROSs is called crosslinking. This is the joining of two molecules that normally wouldn't be joined. The major crosslinked molecule is low-density lipoprotein (LDL). This is the bad cholesterol that everyone is worried about, because these molecules become oxidized (turn rancid) and clump to the insides of arteries and other critical places. The new molecules are now useless and can be deadly if they are allowed to build up. These types of molecules can be found in artery blocking plaques and in the plaques found in the brains of Alzheimer's patients. Another possible cause of these plaques is the sugar glucose, whose effect is discussed in greater detail below.

However, all LDL isn't necessarily bad. Large LDL particles may be harmless, but small LDL particles can be deadly. Cholesterol itself is not bad. The problem starts when cholesterol oxidizes.

However, keep an eye on your level. Very high (or very low) cholesterol indicates your body is out of balance.

Glycation is the term used for crosslinking. Glycation is a chain reaction where sugar and protein or fat molecules tangle up, resulting in deformed or non-functioning molecules. Did you ever notice how old leather cracks? That's caused by molecular cross-linking. The same thing happens to your skin. But what you can't see is the damage it does to you internally.

What else does free radical damage cause? The end results of free radical damage include arthritis, skin aging (wrinkles), cataracts, and blindness. This is on top of increasing your chances of heart disease, cancer stroke, and diabetes.

Okay, so how do we stop this damage from occurring? Diet, exercise, and supplementation can alleviate much of the damage caused by free radicals. Diet can help you control the damage when you eat foods that are high in anti-oxidant molecules, and by eating lower calorie diets. This keeps the mitochondria from working as hard, and reduces the amount of free glucose in your bloodstream. Exercise can control it by giving you greater anti-oxidant potential and better elimination of wastes from your system. Supplementation can control it by giving you additional antioxidant molecules, many of which cannot be obtained in sufficient quantities from diet alone.

We'll get into more detail in Part II.

Other sources of damage to the molecules in your body include smoking, alcohol, toxins, and air and water pollution. The amount of damage to the human body caused by cigarettes and alcohol is truly amazing and a testament to how good our repair systems actually are. Environmental damage from airborne and waterborne chemicals is also a significant concern.

There are most likely other causes of degenerative diseases and aging itself. There are ticking genetic clocks called telomeres in your cells that may cause some of your systems to shut down as you age. The systems that repair damage and keep your metabolism regulated have a drastic effect once removed from action. Some of these key systems include your endocrine system (which regulates hormone release) and your immune system. In addition there are some things that once damaged just can't be repaired very well yet, such as certain organs and joints, and of course your cells.

These other problems and how to control their effects aren't completely understood yet, so we will have to wait for scientists and physicians to make further sense of the aging process.

For example, most scientists' theory of aging holds that aging is a downward spiral consequence of accumulated wear and tear from toxins, free-radical molecules, DNA-damaging radiation, disease and stress. Eventually, your body can't bounce back.

But this theory has recently been challenged by Stanford University Medical School researchers. Their discovery suggests specific genetic instructions drive the aging process.

And Dr. Clifford Steer adds there is evidence that nearly all age-related illnesses involve some degree of damage to DNA. The advances in genetic engineering in the last decade offer great potential for the treatment of acquired or inherited genetic disorders associated with aging. Gene repair has several advantages over other regenerative approaches in terms of potential therapeutic benefit.

If aging is not a cost of unavoidable chemistry but is instead driven by changes in regulatory genes, the aging process, according to many experts, is not inevitable.

According to Dr. Gregory Fahy as stated in *The Future of Aging*, the resources for basic control over aging reside in our own genomes. He believes aging is not only malleable, but even preventable and reversible in mammals.

"Truly effective intervention into aging is likely to require a multiplicity of interventive strategies." There is no question that we are learning how to intervene in the process, and that progress is accelerating.

Dr. Michael West contributes this, also in *The Future of Aging*: "Many researchers quickly ascribe the aging process to entropy, and then just conclude that reversing aging is, for all practical purposes, impossible." He feels these conclusions ignore the fact that the lineage of germ-line cells, unlike their somatic counterparts, replicate in an immortal process of cell division. "This means that these cells must possess sufficient repair mechanisms to allow enough individuals to survive in order to perpetuate their species."

MaxLife supports whatever works and pursues all viable paths.

We will not have to wait long, though. We saw how biomedical knowledge advances exponentially. Every week or two another stunning breakthrough is announced. This section is a practical guide to what you can do now to slow your aging. This might be critical, because the cure for what ails you, including aging, could be literally right around the corner.

Genetics only accounts for 25–35% of how fast we age. The rest is determined by metabolism, which is largely under your control. Anabolic metabolism is the regenerating or restoring activity of your body. Catabolic activity refers to breakdown and degeneration. The rate at which your catabolic activity exceeds your anabolic activity gauges how fast you age. Conversely, the rate at which your anabolic activity exceeds your catabolic activity gauges how fast and how far you reverse your aging process.

For a detailed description and a roadmap on how to help control your aging process, see *The Metabolic Plan* by Stephen Cherniske. The tips in his book focus on boosting your anabolic metabolism and reducing your catabolic metabolism.

So far, we are stuck with aging. But decay is optional. In other words, you mostly control your fate. You don't have to look, feel or act old.

The Economic Case for Health and Longevity

Aging will devastate the modern industrialized world unless something is done to gain control over it.

One problem is, we get sick and die prematurely. People who die at 110 are sick for eight months on average. Those who die between 70 and 80 and are sick for 7 to 8 years and endure triple the medical costs.

According to the Government Accountability Office, by 2020, more than half of all the US federal revenue will go to support the aging population. When interest on the national debt and Medicare are factored in, there will be only eight percent of the total left to pay for other federal programs.

A Harvard University study concluded that 50% of all bankruptcy filings in the U.S. are a direct result of excessive medical expenses. Fifteen percent of America's gross domestic product (GDP) goes to medical care—or $8,233 for each person, according to the Health Data 2012 Report. The overall healthcare cost doubled from 1993 to 2004. Where are medical expenses headed? According to the National Coalition on Health Care, this trend will continue. By 2015, health care spending will soar to $4 trillion, or 20% of GDP.

The boomer generation represents an aging tsunami. In Japan, 40% of the population is projected to be over eighty in a few decades, and we will see similar demographics in the US. If ignored, the economic costs of aging will be five times the cost of the recent trillion dollar mortgage crisis. Meanwhile, Congress tries to figure out ways to tax to pay for the high costs of aging instead of stopping it.

On a personal level, let's conservatively say by incorporating at least one, if not several, tips in this book, you reduce your risk of disease by 50%. That means an additional $4,116 in your pocket—every year.

Now let's talk about how living longer can *make* you money, not just save you money. Let's say the information you get from this book gives you fifteen more healthy years. Do you have any idea what that can do for your net worth? If you compound your portfolio or retirement fund at 10% annual interest (roughly the historical average annual growth of the stock markets, including recessions), in less than fifteen years, you will *quadruple* the value of that account without adding one more penny.

Live longer, and you can become wealthy. How wealthy? Add thirty years, and your account is worth 18 times as much. If you invest your annual $4,116 health expense savings, or even more, it goes up from there.

Before we talk about your seven steps to tomorrow's life extending technologies, let's briefly chat about some of the extreme longevity technologies we are developing.

CHAPTER 4. THE TECHNOLOGIES
THAT WILL SET YOU FREE

A s I mentioned, we're seeing a convergence among biotechnology, information technology and nanotechnology that points straight to open-ended lifespans. I'll briefly cover some examples for you that will give you a peek into this amazing future.

Let's start with biotech.

Strategies for Engineered Negligible Senescence (SENS)

According to one of the world's most notable gerontologists, Dr. Aubrey de Grey, there are only seven fundamental kinds of cell damage that occur in aging (generating such side effects as heart disease, arthritis, diabetes, cancer and more). We believe we will soon have practical solutions for each of them.

Dr. de Grey defines aging as normal metabolism resulting in ongoing damage. That leads to pathology which in turn eventually results in death. It all boils down to accumulating junk (molecular byproducts of the metabolic process). So if we can slow pathology, we have better quality of life for a longer time.

His SENS strategy is to periodically repair the damage to avoid pathology and *not* to interfere with metabolism per se.

Dr. de Grey's approach sees medicine as a branch of engineering. You don't have to know why things go wrong—you just have to be able to fix them. He points out how complex our biochemistry is and how difficult it will be to control it. SENS offers a direct path to reverse much aging-related damage before we learn to control the human aging process. Repairing the damage caused by aging makes understanding those mysteries unnecessary for the time being. As he puts it, "This is no longer a scientific problem, it's an engineering problem."

This would be much like restoring a car or building. As long as you start restoring a car before it deteriorates too badly, you could hypothetically keep it running endlessly.

Dr. de Grey is currently spearheading a ten-year project to reverse aging in elderly mice. Once that proof of concept is demonstrated, the methodologies would be extended to human trials.

Tissue Engineering/Regenerative Medicine

Tissue engineering/regenerative medicine is an emerging multidisciplinary field involving biology, medicine, and engineering that is likely to revolutionize the ways we improve the health and quality of life for millions of people worldwide by restoring, maintaining, or enhancing tissue and organ function. Tissue engineering can perhaps be best defined as creating tissues or organs to replace lost form or function.

It includes using a combination of cells, including stem cells, engineering materials and suitable biochemical factors to improve or replace biological functions. MacArthur and Oreffo defined tissue engineering as "understanding the principles of tissue growth, and applying this to produce functional replacement tissue for clinical use."

Tissue engineering solves problems by using living cells as engineering materials. These could be artificial skin that includes living fibroblasts, cartilage repaired with living cartilage cells, or other types of cells used in other ways.

So far, researchers have been able to grow skin, blood, blood vessels, heart valves, cartilage, bone, noses and ears in the lab. Bladders and tracheas have already been grown and successfully implanted in human patients. Livers and pancreas may be grown as well within five years.

Organs on Demand

As reported in an 11/21/13 Wired.co.uk article, a team of cardiovascular scientists led by Dr. Stuart K. Williams has announced they will be able to 3D print a whole heart from the recipients' own cells within a decade.

The team of more than twenty have already bioengineered a coronary artery and printed the smallest blood vessels in the heart used in microcirculation.

Eventually, they plan to print the whole heart in just three hours, with a further week needed for it to mature outside of the body. Certain parts will need to be printed and assembled beforehand, including the valves and the biggest blood vessels. Williams asserts they are "on schedule" to build the bioficial heart within a decade. The bioprinter is under construction now in Louisville.

Imagine a patient entering the operating room where tissue is removed and regenerative cells isolated. The cells are then mixed with solutions that contain extracellular matrix molecules and other factors and placed in the bioprinter. The bioprinter then prints the heart. Bioengineers have already 3D printed a tiny functioning liver, but the problem is keeping it alive.

The Huffington Post reported on 9/25/13 that dying patients could someday receive a 3D-printed organ made from their own cells rather than wait on long lists for the short supply of organ transplants.

Regenerative medicine pioneers such as Dr. Anthony Atala have already implanted lab-grown skin, tracheas and bladders into patients. In the future, 3D-printing technology will offer both greater speed and computer-guided precision to make replacement skin, body parts and perhaps eventually organs such as hearts, livers and kidneys.

Atala's group previously built lab-grown organs by creating artificial scaffolds in the shape of the desired organ and seeding the scaffold with living cells. They used the technique to grow artificial bladders first implanted in patients in 1999, but spent the last decade building 3D printers that can print both an artificial scaffold and living cells at the same time.

Other labs such as Organovo's think they can bypass the artificial scaffolds by harnessing living cells' tendencies to self-organize. That avoids the challenge of choosing scaffold material that can eventually dissolve without affecting the living cells, but leaves the initial structure of living cells in a delicate position without the supporting scaffold.

Atala's lab recently received U.S. Department of Defense funding for a collaborative project aimed at printing tiny hearts, livers and kidneys to form a connected "body on a chip," ideal for testing possible drugs and the effects of diseases or chemical warfare agents on the human body.

How about BETTER than new? Using 3-D printing tools, scientists at Princeton University have created a functional ear that can "hear" radio frequencies far beyond the range of normal human capability.

Merging electronics with tissue, Princeton University scientists used 3-D printing of cells and nanoparticles with an off-the-shelf printer purchased off the Internet. They followed it by cell culture to combine a small coil antenna with cartilage, creating what they term a bionic ear.

This project is the team's first effort to create a fully functional organ, one that not only replicates a human ability, but extends it using embedded electronics. We look forward to the day when the deaf can hear… better than any human today.

Replacement Stem Cell Therapy

Imagine being seventy and having a thirty-year-old heart, lungs, digestive system, immune system—or even skin and hair!

You could potentially transform your skin or hair to a teenage condition in less than three years. And you may repair your other organs, pending regulatory approval, or be able to bank your organ's stem cells for future use within that same time period.

This technology would isolate your pluripotent stem cells and replace the least viable stem cells with millions of copies of the most perfect or pristine ones.

Pluripotent Stem Cells are master cells, with the ability to grow into any one of the human body's more than 200 cell types.

They are unspecialized (undifferentiated) cells. They retain the ability to divide throughout life and give rise to cells that can become highly specialized and take the place of cells that die or are lost.

Stem cells contribute to the body's ability to renew and repair its tissues. Unlike mature cells, which are permanently committed to their fate, stem cells can both renew themselves as well as create new cells of whatever tissue they belong to (and other tissues).

Stem cell medicine may be the biggest and most promising development in the history of medicine. It holds promise to treat or cure nearly every disease and injury and should have a major impact on aging. So far, researchers have created beating hearts, pituitaries and retinas in animals, and human trials and clinical therapies are taking place around the world.

Currently, adult stem cell therapy using your own stem cells means you get an additional amount of the same stem cells you now carry. Except when the stem cell population is expanded, the cells age with each division. Repopulating your damaged or aged tissue with more cells is an inefficient way to be treated. In addition, giving you more mutated cells raises the question of a cancer risk.

This new technology, once funded, may be able to provide your doctor with the best quality stem cells possible to repopulate your organs. These cells would potentially be amplified a million times or more without aging them or without degradation.

Extensions of this technology would potentially make cells younger when they divide instead of aging them. Cells typically age when they divide.

Several university research teams have been able to take ordinary adult skin stem cells and convert them to look and act exactly like embryonic stem cells. They call these "human iPS cells." Researchers essentially turn back these cells' aging clocks. That means, they would have the raw material that made you, you.

Doctors would basically take some of your cells and transform them to cells that are indistinguishable from the cells you had when you were a baby. Then, when these cells would be injected into your injured, diseased or aged tissue, they could completely repair that tissue. That could be your heart, skin, inner ear, lung, bones or whatever.

You could eventually end up with nearly perfect building blocks to have yourself rejuvenated.

And yet another advancement, In papers published in January, 2014, a Japanese team says it has come up with a surprisingly simple method... exposure to stress... that can make cells that are even more malleable than iPS cells. And they do it faster and more efficiently. On average, 7-8% of those convert to pluripotent cells, already a higher proportion than the roughly 1% conversion rate of iPS cells.

Even now, current stem cell treatments of bad knees using non-optimized adult stem cells typically cost one tenth as much as does standard knee reconstruction surgery. Yet, stem cell therapies appear to last much longer with less pain and down time when compared to standard treatments for the same indication.

Genomics

A California company is capitalizing on a scientific breakthrough and proven scientific and drug discovery techniques to develop therapeutics and diagnostics that will extend and improve quality of life. Their strategy is based on over thirty years of research.

Their chief scientist was the first person in the world to deliberately and significantly postpone aging in experimental organisms. He has created populations of fruit flies that have a lifespan approximately five times that of a normal fruit fly. Although other long-lived experimental organisms exist, his are the only ones that have both increased quality and quantity of life. They are more active for a longer period of time, are more resistant to stress, have more sex, and are generally healthier and more vital.

Researchers in this company are comparing genes in long-lived fruit flies to normal fruit flies and identifying the genes that are different. They found four hundred aging-related genes.

You might wonder why fly studies could be important to human longevity.

You probably don't know that fruit fly genes related to aging are being correlated to their human gene counterparts. They expect to find that about 80-90% of these aging genes will have closely-related genes in humans.

They are now developing diagnostic tests, especially on drugs already marketed (and thus FDA approved) that act on the pathways harboring these genes. Those screened drugs can then be identified that might have anti-aging properties. FDA approval is streamlined. We will soon know which supplements and drugs actually do extend lifespans as well—and which don't.

Genome Reengineering

One of the profound implications of longevity is we are starting to understand our biology as information processes. We have about 20,000 little software programs inside us called genes. These evolved in a different era. One of those programs previously mentioned, called the fat insulin receptor gene, basically says, "Hold onto every calorie, because the next hunting season might not work out so well." We'd like to change that program now.

A new technology called RNA interference puts fragments of RNA inside the cell, as a drug, to inhibit selected genes. It can actually turn genes off by blocking the messenger RNA expressing that gene. When the fat insulin receptor was turned off in mice, the mice ate like horses and stayed slim. They didn't get diabetes, didn't get heart disease, and lived 20% longer. They got the benefit of caloric restriction without moderating how much they eat.

Every major disease and every major aging process has different genes that are used in the expression of these disease and aging processes.

Science and Theology News reported there are thousands of these developments in the pipeline. Our ability to do this is also growing at an escalating rate.

As I said, our genome is simply information. Scrape below the skin and we're flesh, blood and bone. Scrape deeper and we're code. Nobel laureate David Baltimore firmly states: "Biology is today an information science."

We will essentially write biological code to fix or improve our genomes, much like computer scientists have been writing code for years. After all, genomics is simply our ability to read the information encoded in our DNA. Now that we can read it, the next step will be reprogramming it.

One scientist calculated it will take approximately 2,000 man years to write enough biological code for longevity to solve a large part of the aging problem. So, four hundred researchers might be able to accomplish this in five short years plus another 1–2 years to train biotech undergrads or grad students. He also figured it would take only tens of thousands of man years of writing code to reinforce the whole human genome against aging damage and diseases. Implementing the technology may depend on nanomedicine.

Craig Venter, one of the first to sequence the human genome, has already created the first cell with a synthetic genome. He now works at the J. Craig Venter Institute to create synthetic biological organisms.

Nanomedicine

Nanotechnology refers to the control of matter on a scale normally between 1–100 nanometers. One nanometer is a billionth of a meter, or 80,000 times smaller than a human hair.

The oldest nanotechnologist on Earth is Mother Nature—a five billion year-old expert, who has found optimal molecular pathways to solve problems of energy (plant "solar cells" through photosynthesis, or mitochondria synthesis), hardness and elasticity (spider silk) and many more. For a great collection of Nature's nanotechnological solutions, visit the Ask Nature www.asknature. org website.

We work with Robert Freitas, the world's recognized authority on medical applications and implications of molecular nanotechnology, or *nanomedicine*. He has launched a program aimed at developing provable nanomedical life extension technology. This may be the ultimate technology that can cure aging and reverse its effects.

His team constructed a preliminary R&D roadmap, and they have already achieved some of their objectives. They have even established six currently active collaborations.

The technology could have commercially useful early applications. If successful, the company will eventually own a must-have product—indefinite life extension and aging reversal. In a nutshell, nanomedicine could eventually build or repair almost every cell in your body, from the bottom up, atom by atom. At its simplest, aging is a matter of atoms and molecules being out of place. According to nanomedicine scientists Robert Freitas and Ralph Merkle, when we get to the 2020s, we will ultimately have perfected the machines of nanotechnology called nanobots, which are blood cell-sized devices that can go inside your body and brain to perform therapeutic functions, as well as to advance the capabilities of our bodies and brains.

If that sounds too futuristic, Ray Kurzweil points out that we already have blood-cell-size devices that are nano-engineered, working to perform therapeutic functions in animals. For example, one scientist cured Type I diabetes in rats. These nano-engineered devices even identified and destroyed cancer cells. And some of them are now approaching human trials. The 2020's will be the "golden era" of nanomedicine.

Nanomedicine could give us much control of matter and a very efficient way to cure aging damage, injuries and diseases.

Computer/Brain Interface

The human race is extremely resilient and resourceful. We often respond to challenges in creative and unexpected ways.

Scientists such as Dr. Pete Estep recognize that biological evolution is a somewhat haphazard and non-optimizing process that has produced many undesirable artifacts. Among a large number and wide variety of such artifacts, two stand out as the underlying causes of the most pervasive and extreme human suffering: mental and lifespan limitations. Mental inabilities are universal. They ultimately explain our ongoing failures to end human warfare, crime, poverty, and famine, and to completely cure diseases, disabilities, aging and "natural" death. Therefore, these inabilities are even more harmful to humanity than the categories of biomedical dysfunction we currently work to cure.

One plan of this research is to accelerate developing biomedical technologies for overcoming these limitations. It entails taking specific steps toward enhancing memory, learning, and cognition by developing technologies that will give our brains direct links to computers.

How about the prospect of simply thinking of a subject, question or problem and getting an answer directly from the Internet? Imagine how much more efficient our longevity researchers will be with that ability. Science fiction? Maybe. But neuroengineers predict we will have that ability—possibly by 2024 or sooner. In fact, IBM predicts we'll have basic mind-reading computers by the end of 2016. They say we'll be able to use the power of our minds to operate machines.

At the University of Western Ontario, researchers already broke ground. In 2013, they used neuroimaging to read human thoughts via brain activity when they are conveying specific 'yes' or 'no' answers. And brain/machine interfaces have been demonstrated for many years to control external devices using just one's mind.

Some scientists even have longer-term plans aimed at preserving memories. So hang on. We have exciting times ahead.

1,000 Einsteins Will Restore Your Youth – Artificial General Intelligence (AGI)

Where men designed hammers, we now have computers designing computers. This is starting to have a huge impact on aging, because biology is now largely an information technology.

Biology is too complex to be solved without increasingly powerful tools. The ultimate may be AGI.

We now generate much more information than we can process. And there are usually many different ways to interpret any journal article when we do process it. So, you really need an all-encompassing and integrative view in order to accurately interpret each paper as well as to discard erroneous or flawed studies.

PubMed, the database of journal articles, has over 22 million such articles, and more than a million are added every year. Think about how much a person can completely digest; maybe two papers a day, or about 500 papers a year? So with a million coming out and being able to read only 500, or even 1,000, you can see only a tiny fraction of the literature. It's very easy to have a kind of selection bias; to get a small view of the literature, and have that lead you the wrong way. And being human, we forget much of what we read.

So what's a solution? AGI.

The theory and a working prototype for a new kind of computer application (AGI) have been developed. This technology will allow computers to learn, think and respond like humans. They will exhibit *real* intelligence. Such intelligent systems do not exist yet. However, the required knowledge to build them and the proof-of-concept does.

AGI makes up one part of the MaxLife plan to accelerate extreme life extension capabilities. Research aims to create this broad human-like intelligence, rather than narrowly "smart" systems that can operate only as tools for human operators in well-defined domains such as tracking inventory, landing airplanes... or Google!

Yes, as transformative as Google is, its technology is a sophisticated, yet a narrow and relatively "dumb" form of AI. Try to visualize manually searching through millions of web pages to find that special widget you're looking for.

Now imagine machine intelligence with the ability to think and learn on its own as well as humans do. That appears to be in our future. For example, if it gets an education equivalent to a biotech researcher, it could do the research. Two AGI companies estimate a working system could take less than ten years to complete pending funding. Two years later, we could potentially have a fully-trained Ph.D.-equivalent AGI doing research. MaxLife works closely with these two leading companies in this field.

And now that Ray Kurzweil joined forces with Google, Google may have an inside track. And look out for IBM.

Imagine a Ph.D. lab assistant that would have total recall and tirelessly work around the clock. It would be able to download all the data it needs from the Internet almost instantaneously. It could collaborate with humans and other AGI. And then, it could be quickly copied as many times as necessary. That may be what we need to solve something as complex as the biochemical processes that age us.

Imagine unleashing 100,000 AGI researchers. Imagine how much faster they would develop real anti-aging therapies.

We don't need full-scale AGI to make an impact on aging either. Early generations are already showing promise.

The following is a more conservative view of when AGI will become a reality. The former approach is to build machines that do what the brain does, but in different ways. In the following scenario, there is a need to totally understand how our brains work.

Reverse-engineering the human brain so we can simulate it using computers may be a reality by 2030, says Ray Kurzweil, artificial intelligence expert and author of the best-selling book The Singularity is Near. The current controversy, or the more interesting question, is will we have the software or methods of human intelligence? To achieve the methods, the algorithms of human intelligence, there is underway an ambitious project to reverse-engineer the brain. And we are making exponential progress toward that end. According to Kurzweil, if you follow the trends in reverse brain engineering, it's a reasonable conclusion that we will have reverse-engineered the several hundred regions of the brain by the 2020s.

Serious funding is already taking place. The Human Brain Project, an EU Flagship, one billion euro, ten year initiative was announced in 2012. The ultimate aim is to build a working model of the human brain, from neuron to hemisphere level, and simulate it on a supercomputer. Japan is also contributing. Then last year, the United States announced its own initiative, Brain Research through Advancing Innovative Neurotechnologies (BRAIN). The NIH is supposed to fund up to $110 million for research this year.

Let's say you're sixty-five or seventy years old now, though. If so, you might be resigned to saying goodbye to this world. You might figure you have about fifteen more years, because that's what the medical establishment, actuaries, the popular press and friends want you to believe. You might be buying in to the hopelessness and inevitability of a degenerating end to your life. But cheer up, Methuselah. I have another scenario for you.

A Younger Tomorrow—Longevity Escape Velocity

You may not have to stretch it out for twenty, thirty, or more years to turn the corner. What if I told you that, if you can stay healthy for just fourteen more years, you might never die from aging? Well, many respected scientists believe that is the case, and here's why.

In the last five years, science added about a year to your remaining lifespan. That means if you had an eighty-year projected lifespan five years ago, it's now eighty-one. Given reasonable funding, within thirteen years or so, medical technology should add more than one year to your lifespan every year, no matter what your age. In other words, your expected lifespan will continue moving away from you. And since we're adding about two months per year now and increasing as we progress, during those fourteen years, we could add about another five to seven years. Anti-aging experts call this your Longevity Escape Velocity.

That's one reason I am convinced many of us will be enjoying fantastic unforgettable sex on our 100th birthdays, while others will be distant memories in their former partners' minds.

Is Escape Velocity an excuse to slack off? Absolutely not! It's every reason to give you hope and to improve your healthy habits. Don't forget, if actuaries are correct about your expected remaining lifespan, about half the people your age will die before then. So don't be "seduced" by breakthroughs you believe will save you from yourself. This is the worst time in history to roll dice with your life.

Want to follow our progress, including the newest technology breakthroughs? Then go to www.MaxLife.org/sssbook.

Now that you have a little background, let's take a look at how soon we think all these great plans could be completed once funding begins.

MaxLife Aggressive Age Reversal Program

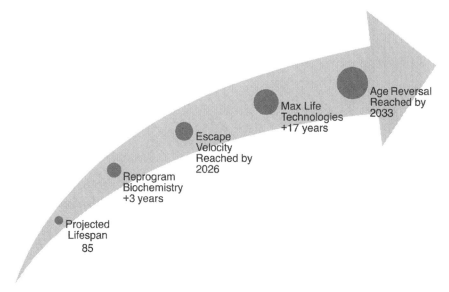

Hypothetical Healthy Seventy-Five-Year-Old Male

*About half the seventy-five year olds will die before age eighty-five and half after. Sixty-five year olds can expect to die by age eighty-one without intervention. Females live longer on average.

How realistic is this model? Maybe it's slightly conservative. In a study of risk factors that may be part of the 65–75% of human lifespan variation not attributable to genetics, Brigham & Women's Hospital researchers estimated that a seventy-year-old man who did not smoke and had normal blood pressure and weight, no diabetes and exercised two to four times per week had a 54% probability of living to age ninety.

That means we could add five or six years to the projected lifespan in the above illustration. (If you're older than seventy and have the same profile, you would have a better than average chance of living beyond ninety, since the older you are the longer you typically live.)

However, if he had adverse factors, his probability of living to age 90 was reduced to these following amounts: sedentary lifestyle—44%, hypertension—36%, obesity—26%, smoking—22%, three factors combined—14%, and five factors combined—4%. As you can see, the more action you take now, the better your odds. Don't ever think it's too late to start taking control over your rate of aging. Never accept that you are just getting too old. You're not. As long as you're alive, you can improve.

We know people are reversing their biological ages by as much as twenty-five years through the seven simple steps outlined in this book. Those with the worst habits have more to potentially reverse, assuming they are not too far gone. That's why I think it's possible for a sixty-five-year-old diabetic with arthritis, high blood pressure and an out-of-balance cholesterol profile to have that unforgettable sex on his or her 100th birthday!

But to improve your odds at any age or condition, you'll need to keep yourself from deteriorating too badly for repair when it's available. Making MaxLife's seven simple steps a routine part of your life could bridge you to tomorrow's life-giving medicine. Read on to see how.

PART II

Seven Steps You Can Take Now to Put Extreme Longevity Odds on Your Side

Seventy-one million Americans have some form of "silent killer" cardiovascular disease. If you're over fifty, the chances are you are one of them. You just don't know how healthy you are based on how you feel. You could feel great now and be dead tomorrow.

Fortunately, the vast majority of heart disease is avoidable by incorporating the information you hold in your hands. You start with exercise and diet. Inactive people are almost twice as likely to get heart disease as active people.

Medicine largely ignores the fact that too many people *get* cancer in the first place, and concentrates on treating it when it strikes. Much cancer, like heart disease, can be avoided by the steps outlined in this book as well. Cancer looks for the weakest cells in your body to attack. Then it silently grows into full-blown cancer. These cells can be weakened by stress, toxins, poor diet, vitamin deficiencies and lack of regular exercise.

Each of the next seven chapters delivers information, advice and tips on the easiest way for you to lock in enhanced energy, vitality, strength, health and longevity.

Taking care of yourself pushes you farther out into the future, closer to the day when new life extending technologies are developed. Funding the technologies pulls their development closer to the present. The push/pull combination increases your chances, along with millions of others, to live long instead of dying prematurely. Many people taking an active role in this push/pull process could get a sneak preview and a jump start on some of the emerging treatments.

Welcome aboard the Longevity Express. The next seven chapters show you how to ensure you reach your destination.

Chapter 5. Step 1—Nutrition

"Nothing tastes as great as being healthy and fit feels."

All seven steps are vital. If I were forced to pick one above all though, it would be Nutrition a.k.a Diet, edging out Exercise. However, this assumes you are at least moderately active, and it's only your starting point, not your end-point. Exercise is more effective than most *standard* models of healthy diets.

Nutrition is critical, because the largest volume of chemicals to which your internal organs are exposed come from your food. The most powerful weapon you currently have for fighting the ravages of aging is a healthy diet.

A good diet lowers risk of death from all causes.

Some foods can be absolutely toxic, especially in the Western part of the world. For millions of years, the balance between oxidants and antioxidants was pretty well balanced. But starting about 10,000 years ago, we got away from the Paleolithic, hunting-gathering diets that consisted of about 70% mostly raw fruits and vegetables, started growing our food, and got away from eating a wide variety of raw foods. Then we gradually started cooking more and processing food as well. Cooking destroys many vital nutrients, and overcooking can create carcinogens.

The U.S. government reports genetic mutations are responsible for an estimated 6,000 diseases, including all cancers. Researchers believe if this one factor were eliminated, humans would routinely live to 100 years and beyond. In fact, if every cell's DNA replaced itself perfectly during cell division, we would be more likely to reach a lifespan of approximately 120 years.

But they don't, thanks in large part to the way we cook our food. Well-done, grilled, fried or barbecued meats instead of baking or stewing at moderate temperatures are mutating your genes. Eating poultry with skin does the same.

Key Points Regarding the Effects of Cooking on Food and Health

> ➤ Much of food's life force is greatly depleted or destroyed when it is overcooked. The bioelectrical energy field is altered and greatly depleted, and has been graphically demonstrated with Kirlian photography.

> ➤ Fiber in plant foods is broken down into a soft, passive substance that loses its broom-like and magnetic cleansing quality in the intestines.

> ➤ Nutrients, like vitamins, minerals, and amino acids are depleted, destroyed, and altered. The degrees are simply a matter of temperature, cooking method, and time. For example, if you cook raw broccoli in the microwave, with a little water added to it, it can lose up to 97% of the antioxidant benefits that the food contained prior to being microwaved. If you steam broccoli, it will lose less than 11% of its nutrients.

> ➤ Up to 50% of the protein may be coagulated when cooked. Much of it may be rendered unusable.

> ➤ The interrelationship of nutrients is altered from its natural synergistic makeup.

> ➤ Overcooking creates unusable waste material, which has a cumulative congesting and clogging effect on your body and is a burden to the natural eliminative processes of your body.

> ➤ Many enzymes present in raw foods are destroyed at temperatures as low as 118 degrees Fahrenheit. Some of these enzymes are important for optimum digestion.

> ➤ Some raw food is more easily digested and may pass through the digestive tract in a half to a third of the time it takes for some cooked food.

> ➤ After eating some cooked foods, there is a rush of white blood cells towards the digestive tract, leaving the rest of the body less protected by the immune system. From the point of view of the immune system, the body is being invaded by a foreign (toxic) substance when some cooked food is eaten.

And it goes on and on. In general, your aging process is accelerated by too much cooked food. People who lean toward raw food often become biologically and visibly younger.

MaxLife recommends you obtain a minimum of 30–50% of your food as uncooked. Vegetable juicing and a salad at lunch will easily put you at that volume.

The Downside of Raw Food

Many people with poor digestion don't handle raw foods or beans very well though. The higher proportion of nutrients in raw food is useless if the food can't be digested, absorbed and assimilated.

Raw foods also have a higher percentage of bacteria and parasites, such as most commercial chicken and a good deal of beef and pork. Although some raw food is digested more efficiently, many vegetables, unless juiced, are harder to digest when raw. The phytates or anti-factors in grains also bind up minerals, making them unavailable to the human body, a probable reason why most grain has traditionally been fermented or sprouted rather than eaten raw or simply ground into flour.

Many beans and legumes, especially raw soybeans, lentils, black-eyed peas, peanuts and mung beans, also contain trypsin inhibitors, which block key digestive enzymes.

Raw sprouts, green onions and lettuce may be sources of food-borne illness, so wash these and all raw foods thoroughly before you eat them. And raw (sprouted) kidney beans and rhubarb can be poisonous.

While cooking can destroy vitamins, it helps with the absorption of carotenoids such as beta-carotene and other nutrients. This is why most nutritionists recommend a mix of some cooked food with raw products.

So there are tradeoffs in each case. Ultimately it comes down to each individual situation—and a matter of balance.

A great way to discover what works best for you is to read *Dr. Mercola's Total Health Program*. It's much more than just a cookbook. This food and lifestyle guide recommends all the real, whole, healthiest foods—both lightly cooked and raw—from the right sources, in the right proportions, in a comprehensive program that is all about balance. You get key information, tools and recipes that let you access and identify your own personal metabolic type. It helps you learn how to listen to your body, to fine-tune your diet to the foods and macronutrient ratios, the ratios of fat, protein and carbohydrates that are precisely what you need.

Instead of thinking raw foods versus cooked foods, focus on getting a *balance* of raw and cooked foods, depending upon the season, climate, your health, level of spiritual evolution, etc. Dr. Mercola's program makes choosing easy for you.

Some general cooking rules are to cook at low temperatures, lightly steam vegetables, stir fry when you fry, and poach your eggs.

Tickle Your Taste Buds with Raw Foods

I understand how challenging maintaining a raw food diet can be. Let's face it. Processed food is engineered to taste good. That's one reason it's so easy to get hooked on it. As far as taste goes, ice cream beats spinach hands down.

If you want to do anything regularly, it's got to taste or feel good. So what's the easiest way to adhere to a largely raw foods diet? The answer is simple and enjoyable. Green smoothies. Since fiber mitigates the sugar in fruits, I recommend smoothies over juice. Juicing eliminates the fiber unless you use a fiber preserving blender such as a Vitamix.

"Greens are the only living thing in the world that can transform sunshine into the food that all creatures can consume," points out Victoria Boutenko. She goes on to explain in her book, *Green Smoothie Revolution,* that without green leaves, there would be no [complex] life on our planet. She also reminds us that greens contain all the essential minerals, vitamins except for B12, and amino acids that humans need for optimal health. And best of all, she discloses how to make the healthiest foods taste even better than the unhealthiest.

Integrate superfoods into your diet too. Superfoods are almost always eaten raw. They have a dozen or more unique properties, not just one or two. Superfoods can turn your health and your life around. They are nature's most perfect foods, and for the most part, are delicious. Learn more about them from David Wolfe's book, *Superfoods: The Food and Medicine of the Future.*

When a Value Meal Isn't

One day, my friend John Lustyan found himself driving by Whole Foods and feeling like a snack. He pulled in and spent 75 cents on a big, delicious, organic Fuji apple. Munching away on it, with the radio on in his car, he heard an all too familiar commercial for a 99-cent meal.

He said there was a time he might have thought: "Darn, I could've gotten a full meal for 24 cents more."

Knowing what he does today, he thought: "We've all bought the ingredients to make a taco or burger using real meat, lettuce, and cheese. We know how much it costs. Yet, this company pays for:

- The ingredients,
- Meal packaging,
- Trays, utensils and napkins,
- Tables and chairs,

- Their cooks and servers,

- Cooking & refrigeration equipment,

- The restaurant rent,

- All their utilities and...

- Daily advertising in print, on TV and the radio, like he'd just heard."

So he asked himself... and hoped other listeners were doing the same: "What in the world are they doing with, and adding to, naturally wholesome food—making it worth so little—that they still make a profit by selling it at 99 cents?"

Processed Food

Processed food is enormously profitable. It is big business at its worst (and this is coming from a free-market enthusiast). When it comes to deciding who to believe, follow the money. The food giants spend billions on advertising to steer you toward their products and away from whole natural foods. Their lobbies spend small fortunes to influence your politicians as well. The result— Americans are the fattest society in history.

So food can be a double-edged sword. With every bite, you either pay a price or reap a reward.

How poisonous is your diet? Did you know bad diets can do more damage to you than smoking (and smoking kills over half of all smokers)? Imagine how your life can come to a grinding halt once you suffer a serious stroke or get cancer. If you mentally classify processed foods as "poisons," instead of viewing dangerous foods as treats, visualize the damage done to your DNA with each bite. Eating sensibly reduces disease risk in people of all ages, so it's never too late to start eating well. My best advice is to regard many popular foods as poisons that will cause you unimaginable suffering and premature death.

You obviously need food to sustain, strengthen and energize your life. Whether it enriches you or kills you is your decision. And you don't need to endure a painful diet for optimal health. The Express is all about having a long full life while enjoying the ride. You can easily elevate your mind, body and spirit because you *want* to take the steps, not because you have to. It's all a matter of learning a few basics.

Once you understand the difference between nourishment and deadly food cravings, your food choices will generally be healthy, since you cherish your life and your looks. Rather than using food to extinguish cravings like you would a campfire, eat vibrant, raw living food to stoke your fire.

So here's your exercise: Hesitate between your urge to eat and actually eating. Consider your rewards or consequences with each temptation. As your awareness grows, it won't take conscious thought at all. You will naturally and effortlessly gravitate toward life-enhancing food, since we get uncomfortable when our actions conflict with our values. Eventually, you will be so used to running on high grade fuels that nothing else will satisfy you.

We tend to get away with a lot of things when we're young that we can't get away with as we age. The young typically get away with bad food, although kids are getting much worse now. They are actually getting Type 2 diabetes. Millions of children are now affected. You never saw that twenty years ago.

So what can we do about it?

Breakthrough Discovery – How to Stop Your Aging Now

I have a good friend, Dr. Michael Rose, who is a preeminent evolutionary biologist with thirty-four years of research under his belt. The specialty from which he has attained international acclaim is, you guessed it, longevity.

Fifteen years of his research were devoted to proving aging *cannot* be stopped. He finished that phase of his research early in 2010 and came to the surprising conclusion that… he was wrong. Yes, he says, according to his conclusions, aging *can* be stopped. And he draws on his lab's thousands of papers and calculations to support it from the standpoint of adaptation to our diets over millions of years.

The best part is Dr. Rose says you can stop your rate of degeneration right now, today. Anyone can. I believe this is the single most important thing you can do for your longevity, bar none.

For details, please see Appendix A

Caloric Restriction

How much should you eat? Generally speaking, the less you eat, the healthier you'll be. And probably the longer you'll live. But before we generalize ourselves into the hospital, let's dig deeper.

We know calorie counting is key. But it's even MORE important to look at the source of the calories than counting them. Sure, you get fat because you eat too much. But as you're seeing in this chapter, you get fat and sick from eating the wrong kind of calories.

Here's just one example of what overeating can do to you.

Eating too many calories at once overloads your bloodstream with fats and sugars long after your meal. That causes severe oxidative and inflammatory damage to your inner arterial walls. That's just one meal. Imagine the cumulative damage caused by chronically overeating. No wonder cardiovascular disease is our number one killer.

Of all the techniques that have been tried on mammals in an attempt to slow the process of aging and extend the maximum life span, the only one that works definitively in many mammals is caloric restriction. This technique has been used on mice, rats, and most recently monkeys. It consists of reducing the total number of calories ingested by an animal by 30%. This technique has resulted in an average of a 15% and as high as a 40% increase in the maximum lifespan of rodents. The monkey studies are conflicting regarding extending maximum lifespan but consistent when it comes to health and appearance.

The calorically restricted monkeys looked and acted younger. And most of them had healthier hearts and immune systems and lower rates of diabetes, cancer and fewer age-related diseases than the control monkeys. That's true for humans who practice CR too.

There's more evidence that humans experience the exact same type of effects from caloric restriction as animals do. Okinawa natives eat about 40% fewer calories than Americans and live about 7% longer and are 75% more likely to retain their cognitive ability. Both animals and humans show lower blood glucose, lower cholesterol and decreased blood pressure while undergoing caloric restriction. These factors may be prime mechanisms of life extension in animals and could very possibly lead to slightly longer maximum lifespans in humans.

But we're endlessly inundated with temptations to eat unhealthy calories. You may enjoy the taste and convenience of refined sugar, saturated and modified fats, simple carbohydrates and processed foods, but your body is designed for something far different.

A Cornell University study confirmed people are powerless to resist overeating if foods are visible and convenient. Another study concluded specific changes occur in our brains when we're tempted with foods. That's one reason it can be so tough to eat healthy.

Like most of us, do you lack willpower? If so, simply keep junk food out of your house. Know this: People eat for entertainment, not for nutrition. When you grocery shop, shop on a full stomach to keep from being tempted by every junk food goodie on the shelves.

Do You Need to Starve Yourself?

Okay, so are we saying we should all go out and reduce our calories by 30%? Not necessarily. It's a tough way to live. I recommend about a 10% reduction in calories from the suggested amount of calories for your optimum weight, gender age and activity level. That equates to about 2,000-2,400 calories a day on average for an adult instead of close to 3,000 calories consumed daily by most Americans (according to a USDA General Survey). So for this example, you would reduce your intake by 200 calories or so.

You can get very fast benefits once you start restricting calories, even up to late mid-age. Your benefits revert if you stop though. Do not reduce the number of calories you eat if you are over the age of seventy and close to your ideal weight, as elderly people have difficulty absorbing enough of their food as it is. If you are overweight you should be reducing your caloric intake anyway.

If you are serious about proceeding with caloric restriction, we suggest you follow the advice of Dr. Roy Walford, one of the pioneers in this field. He wrote an excellent book on the subject, *The Anti-Aging Plan*. His website, www.walford.com, contains excellent diet software.

Reducing calories by 30% is a Spartan diet, it takes discipline to adhere to it, and there may be no more benefits than a 10% reduction would give you. One easier way to cut your calories is to simply use smaller plates and to keep the rest of the food out of sight. You can easily cut your calories by 20% this way without feeling deprived.

For convenience, you might want to forget about counting calories and simply focus on portions. Each portion of protein and carbohydrates at each meal should be about the size of your palm. Since fat is much denser, and since fewer calories should come from fat in most cases, keep your portion to about one-quarter to one-third the size of your palm. Reduce those portions slightly for caloric restriction.

As Dr. Walford and others have pointed out, what type of food you eat is also very important when practicing caloric restriction. You must still eat a fully nutritionally balanced meal. This means you should eat foods that are low in calories and high in essential vitamins, minerals and nutrients.

Does this mean you have to be a fanatic and give up some of your best pleasures of life? Not at all. It just means you should be aware of the consequences of overeating and of an unhealthy diet. If you're not able or willing to change your diet overnight, start with one day a week. Then two. Work your way up to five or six and indulge one or two days if you absolutely must. Otherwise, with the way science is charging forward, you may be eating yourself into missing the super longevity train.

When it comes to overeating and unhealthy diets, be aware of your choice between short-term gratification and long-term satisfaction, health and longevity. This means you should apply the same sensibilities to your health that you should apply to your job, business or finances.

Having said that, there is light at the end of the tunnel for those who want the benefits of caloric restriction (CR) without cutting calories drastically. New supplements and drugs are being developed called CR mimetics. They send the same messages to your genes that cutting calories does. So you could get the same benefits from these compounds as you get from eating less. Think of this as having your cake and eating it too.

Each bite of food contains hundreds or thousands of individual chemicals that affect a wide range of your bodily functions. Let's talk a bit about how carbohydrates, proteins and fats influence your body's biochemistry, so you have a better understanding of how your various foods affect you.

Carbohydrates

Carbohydrates are your main fuel source and are the most consumed nutrients in the world. They fall into three major categories: sugars, complex carbohydrates and fiber.

Simply put, carbohydrates are fiber or non-fiber. Fiber is good for you, and non-fiber carbs are bad. When you eat a non-fiber carbohydrate, it turns into sugar.

Your body needs to break down the sugars into a simple sugar called glucose so your body can use it as fuel. Your body stores the glucose it doesn't use in a form called glycogen. When your blood glucose drops too low, glycogen is converted to more glucose. If you use up all your glycogen, your body starts breaking down your muscle tissue to get more glucose. Two major hormones that regulate this process are insulin and glucagon. When your blood sugar levels rise typically after you eat carbohydrates, insulin signals your body to store your excess glucose. Glucagon has the opposite duty. It signals your muscles and liver to convert glycogen back to glucose to dump back into your bloodstream. Diabetics have abnormally high blood glucose levels.

A high simple carbohydrate diet has been implicated as being a factor in heart disease, cancer, diabetes and a whole host of other problems. If you are on a low carbohydrate diet, be sure to supplement with at least thirty grams of a high quality fiber.

The glycemic index is a measure of how much foods elevate blood sugar levels. Simple sugars have a high glycemic index. These are the foods that are most prone to triggering diabetes over time and increase your storage of body fat. Larger, more complex carbohydrates have a low glycemic index, because they cause a gradual increase in blood glucose levels.

To reduce your chances of diabetes and obesity, eat low glycemic foods like nuts, seeds, fruits and non-starchy vegetables. If you insist on eating grains, eat only whole grains (especially barley).

Stay away from high glycemic index and glycemic load foods such as sugar, white bread, cookies, cakes, candy, soft drinks and jams. Freshly ground cinnamon can reduce the glycemic index of a meal by up to 29%. Take up to four grams with any given meal (about 1.5 teaspoons) to lower your blood glucose as well as your LDL cholesterol and triglycerides. Since it could have a blood thinning effect, limit your consumption to four grams a day.

But there's more to the story than glycemic index. The glycemic index compares the potential of foods containing the same amount of carbohydrate to raise blood glucose. But the amount of carbohydrates you eat also affects blood glucose levels and insulin responses.

The glycemic load of a food is calculated by multiplying the glycemic index by the amount of carbohydrates in grams in a food and dividing the total by 100. The concept of glycemic load was developed by scientists to simultaneously describe the quality (glycemic index) and quantity of carbohydrates in your meal or diet. Your body's insulin response is affected more by a food's glycemic load than by the glycemic index.

See the table below for the glycemic index and glycemic load values of popular foods. Foods with higher glycemic index values are at the top of the table (worse for you), while foods with lower index values (better for you) are at the bottom. To find the glycemic index, glycemic load or name of individual foods, go to www. glycemicindex.com, and click on GI Data-base.

Glycemic Index and Glycemic Load Values for Selected Foods (Relative to Glucose)				
Food	Glycemic Index (Glucose=100)	Serving size	Carbohydrate per serving (g)	Glycemic Load per serving
Dates, dried	103	2 oz	40	42
Cornflakes	81	1 cup	26	21
Jelly beans	78	1 oz	28	22
Puffed rice cakes	78	3 cakes	21	17
Russet potato (baked)	76	1 medium	30	23
Doughnut	76	1 medium	23	17
Green Peas	75	1 cup	22	6
Soda crackers	74	4 crackers	17	12
White bread	73	1 large slice	14	10
Table sugar (sucrose)	68	2 tsp	10	7
Pancake	67	6" diameter	58	39
White rice (boiled)	64	1 cup	36	23
Brown rice (boiled)	55	1 cup	33	18
Carrots	47	1 cup	12	4
Spaghetti, white; boiled 10–15 min	44	1 cup	40	18
Oranges, raw	42	1 medium	11	5
Rye, pumpernickel bread	41	1 large slice	12	5
Spaghetti, white; boiled 5 min	38	1 cup	40	15

Pears, raw	38	1 medium	11	4
Apples, raw	38	1 medium	15	6
All-Bran™ cereal	38	1 cup	23	9
Spaghetti, whole wheat; boiled	37	1 cup	37	14
Skim milk	32	8 fl oz	13	4
Lentils, dried; boiled	29	1 cup	18	5
Kidney beans, dried; boiled	28	1 cup	25	7
Pearled barley; boiled	25	1 cup	42	11
Cashew nuts	22	1 oz	9	2
Peanuts	14	1 oz	6	1

Source: Jane Higdon, Ph.D., Linus Pauling Institute, Oregon State University

Proteins

Proteins maintain your body's normal structure and function. Proteins are the building blocks of your tissues, enzymes, DNA, hemoglobin and antibodies. Your body's proteins are made up of twenty amino acids. Your body makes twelve, and you need to get the other eight, the "essential amino acids" from the food you eat. If you don't get enough of these eight, your body can't repair itself, your immune system suffers, your metabolism slows down, and so do you.

If one amino acid out of twenty is missing, or is in short supply, then that limits your protein synthesis. So what are your best sources of essential amino acids? Whey protein tops the list, followed by eggs (I suggest omega-3 enriched eggs). You can accomplish the same thing by combining lentils and rice, legumes or vegetables and grains, legumes and vegetables and nuts and mushrooms and vegetables. But if super longevity is your goal, eliminate grains altogether, as well as dairy and legumes. That means egg protein may be a better choice than whey.

If you shy away from animal products, or even if you don't, try spirulina. This algae is one of nature's most perfect foods. It is a complete protein source and has the highest concentration of protein found in any food. AFA blue-green algae from Klamath Lake is nearly as good. Try both.

Hempseed also contains all the essential amino acids, and in a high concentration. Plus it provides you with all the essential fatty acids in a perfect ratio. This is a true superfood for vegetarians and meat eaters alike.

Proteins do not spike your blood sugar levels like carbohydrates do. They are also more satiating and increase your metabolism more than carbohydrates and fats.

A group of scientists and physicians have been very vocal in advocating what the mainstream media and the medical establishment calls a "high protein diet." This group includes Dr. Robert Atkins, *Atkins Diet*; Dr. Barry Sears, *Zone Diet*; Drs. Andrews, Balart, and Bethea, *Sugar Busters*; and Drs. Mary and Michael Eades, *Seed Power*.

None of these diets is really extremely high in protein; they are just lower in carbohydrates than what the USDA has been recommending for the past thirty years. This group and Dr. Walford are essentially all saying the same thing—simple carbohydrates can kill!

After a thorough review of the literature, it becomes clear that these people are right. Anyone who is saying 60%+ of your diet should be carbohydrates is dead wrong (pun intended) unless they are made up exclusively of high-fiber complex carbohydrates found in foods such as raw vegetables and fruits, and if you are a carbohydrate nutritional type. If you're interested in losing weight or staying healthy, find out what your type is. You can use your favorite search engine to find websites that will give you online tests to see where you stand. Search for "metabolic type testing." Your anti-aging physician may be able to give you a more accurate test in his or her office.

Fats

Fat is not the villain many make it out to be. All your trillions of cell membranes are made of fat. Next to water, fat is the most abundant substance in your body. Ideally, your body weight should be made up of 10–20% fat. Women typically carry a higher percentage of body fat than men.

You may have heard of the different kinds of fat including the "good" fats and the "bad" fats. We often hear how bad saturated fats are for us. But nutritional typing predicts that one-third of people will do very well on low saturated fat diets (which supports the studies showing they work), but another one-third of people need high saturated fat diets to stay healthy. Saturated fats actually play crucial roles in many body functions and should account for about 20–25% of the fats you consume on average. Get these from low-fat meats like organic poultry, coconut oil and lean red meat from grass-fed/free-range animals.

Polyunsaturated fats, so called "good" fats, help to reduce inflammation and decrease serum cholesterol. Find these omega-3 fatty acids in fish and fish and krill oil, flax oil, walnuts and algae. Polyunsaturated fats are normally liquid at room temperature, and saturated fats are usually solid.

Commercial food processors often solidify polyunsaturated fats through a hydrogenation process to increase their products' shelf life. These are called trans-fats and are linked to cancer, atherosclerosis, diabetes, obesity, immune system dysfunction and—well, you get the idea. You'll find these trans-fats in processed packaged foods like chips, baked goods, candy and margarine.

Then we have monounsaturated fats. They increase your good cholesterol (HDL) and lower your bad cholesterol (LDL). Find these in olives, pure virgin olive oil, nuts and avocados.

Why Obesity is Becoming Epidemic

Eating fat will not make you fat.

Unless you're a carb nutritional type, eating excessive carbs and sugar is virtually guaranteed to pack on the pounds. Why?

Because your cells need fuel to function and they can get their fuel in the form of sugar or fat. But here's the kicker. Your body will burn all of the available sugar first before it turns to burning fat. So let's say you eat loads of pasta, sugar, bread, baked goods, crackers, cookies and countless other carbs. Your body doesn't know how to handle all that sugar, so it continues turning it into fat to get it out of your bloodstream.

For a while, you'll keep gaining weight. This is actually in response to your cells keeping you alive by turning the excess sugar into fat. Eventually, though, even your fat stores can get filled up. This is why people who become obese almost always end up with diabetes; there's no place left to store the excess sugar as fat, so it stays in your bloodstream, driving your insulin levels up.

The solution? Eat less carbs and sugar, and eat more healthy fats.

This way, your body can easily burn the sugar that you do eat and continues to be adept at burning fat as well. You'll stay leaner and healthier, and you'll feel fuller, too.

We all need some fat, but some of us need upwards of 50% of our diet in the form of fat, while others need as little as 10%. The distinction depends on your nutritional, or metabolic type.

One of the best benefits of learning your nutritional type is you don't have to worry about counting calories or fat grams. Instead you focus on eating the right proportion of carbs, fats and protein for your body. It's a much more natural, intuitive way of eating. And you'll know when you've found the right ratio for you, because you'll feel wonderful.

Why Diabetes is Becoming Epidemic

Some of the most damaging groups of substances we are exposed to on a daily basis are starches and refined sugars such as sucrose, fructose, glucose, dextrose and corn syrup. Our metabolism was just not designed to handle the tremendous amount of nutrient-free calories (i.e., sugar, starches, and to some degree fat) that the typical American diet has in it. The majority of those calories come from refined sugar (sweets, soft drinks, etc.) and starches (bread and pasta).

Excess sugar and starch cause multiple assaults to your system. First, as we discussed, high blood sugar causes excess insulin release. Of the two hormones that control the amount of sugar in your blood stream—insulin and glucagon, insulin causes sugar to be taken into the cells, while glucagon causes it to be released. By eating excess carbohydrates, you put your blood sugar control system onto a dangerous roller coaster ride. Up, down, up, down—after repeated bouts of this, your system will crash. The result is Type 2 diabetes, which is becoming more and more prevalent.

There's more. People with diabetes are twice as likely to have arthritis. In fact, more than half of the U.S. adults diagnosed with diabetes also have arthritis. That puts them in a double bind, as the pain in their joints keeps them from getting the exercise they need to keep both diseases at bay.

Diabetics are unable to take up sugar efficiently, because their cells no longer respond to insulin. A nasty side effect of this process is that your body begins producing way too much insulin to try and overcome the unresponsiveness of your cells. So now you have high insulin and high blood sugar, which causes all kinds of damage to your arteries. This includes higher cholesterol in your blood, more useless molecules being made by sticking to the excess sugar (crosslinking) which clogs your arteries, the production of oxidized molecules, and the release of the hormone cortisol which causes tissue breakdown.

Insulin also causes excess sugar to be converted to fat. Want to lose weight? Stay away from white flour and sugar.

We also know sugar depresses the immune system. The root of all disease, common cold or cardiovascular disease, osteoporosis or cancer, is at the molecular and cellular level. And insulin is probably going to be involved in almost every aging disease, if not totally controlling it.

Insulin is that important.

Some of us are less susceptible to the perils of sugar and starch than others. Starch in general does not cause diabetes according to a study by Dr. Richard Johnson, the chief of the division of kidney disease and hypertension at the University of Colorado, and author of *The Sugar Fix*. The new appreciation is that if you have your uric acid level checked and have a level of 4 for men or 3.5 for women, you probably are at a low risk for fructose toxicity and can be more liberal with your intake.

The higher your uric acid is though, the more you need to limit fructose to about 16 grams a day, or even avoid it until your uric acid level normalizes.

Even with a healthy uric acid level, I suggest avoiding all foods with added fructose like the plague. A growing lineup of scientific studies is demonstrating that consuming high-fructose corn syrup is the fastest way to trash your health. It is now known without a doubt that sugar in your food, in all its myriad of forms, is taking a devastating toll.

And fructose in any form, including high-fructose corn syrup (HFCS) and crystalline fructose, is the worst of the worst!

To replace those high-calorie, low-nutrient carbohydrates you were consuming before, eat lots of raw fruit and vegetables. Some fruits that have been discovered to be particularly good for their anti-aging properties are blueberries, pomegranates, bilberries, strawberries, purple grapes, and tomatoes (Yes, tomatoes are technically fruits, not vegetables). Since fruits contain natural fructose, I suggest you eat more veggies than fruit.

The deeper and richer the colors of your fruits and vegetables, the more nutritional value they have for you. If your meals look like rainbows, you're on the right track. Why all the fuss about color? Because loads of scientific studies have shown the natural pigments that give fruits and veggies their vibrant colors offer remarkable health benefits. A major class of compounds in this category is the flavonoids.

Flavonoids are powerful antioxidants that are linked with health benefits including protection from cancer, heart disease, dementia, diabetes, stroke and more.

Fruits with rich colors, especially deep blue or purple, tend to have high concentrations of anthocyanins, one of nature's most potent classes of flavonoids. And get this. In case you haven't heard, dark chocolate and red wine are also rich sources of flavonoids. A study at University Hospital Zurich showed 6 grams of dark chocolate a day reduces risks of heart disease and stroke by 39%. Take it easy though. Too much dark chocolate will overdose you with sugar and saturated fat. Limit yourself to 7.5 grams of dark chocolate a day. More than two glasses of red wine a day works against you due to excess alcohol and sugar. Moderation is the word of the day if you must indulge.

Strawberries have high concentrations of ellagic acid, another antioxidant that has been shown to protect rats against many age-related defects. The molecule lycopene in tomatoes is yet another powerful antioxidant.

If you do eat simple carbohydrates, take some high-grade protein with it to reduce its damage by about half. Don't beat yourself up and worry about eating a hamburger, ice cream or pizza once in a while if it gives you pleasure. But making it a habit will undermine your health and shorten your life.

On the flip side, when you plan your meal or snack, visualize yourself as being healthier and slimmer. Then concentrate on your food while eating, and reward yourself mentally when you make your healthy choices.

Eat a Wide Variety of Fresh or Frozen Produce—and Lots of It

The quarter of the population eating the fewest fruits and vegetables has over three times as much heart disease as the quarter of the population that eats the most. Eat a minimum of six servings of fresh vegetables per day. This isn't as much as it seems. One serving equals only one-half cup or one cup if they are leafy vegetables. A good rule of thumb is to stay with brightly colored veggies. And eat a wide variety—mostly raw and organic, if possible.

Also add one to three servings of fresh fruit per day. Again have a wide variety—and again, raw and organic if possible. Buying local produce may be more important than buying organic, since freshness is so important. You're better off buying fresh, vibrant, conventionally grown produce than wilted organic.

Stay away from white potatoes, too. Your body reacts to them like it reacts to white bread. Increasing vegetables and fruits from two servings to only five servings a day can cut the incidence of many cancers in half. That's only two and one-half cups. Consider getting a Vita Mix. It's like a kitchen in one appliance and is the best juicer on the market.

Make sure you get your money's worth from your juicer. Drink five glasses of fresh juiced fruits and veggies every week. I combine several fruits and veggies in my drinks, changing the mix each time. As an alternative, you might get a high quality "green drink" in powder form. Mix with water and drink every day. There are lots of good ones on the market. I have yet to find one that is Paleo.

The human body evolved with a diet that was high in fruits and vegetables. If you fight nature with your diet, your health and energy level will tank. People are shocked at how much better they feel after substituting high-fiber foods for fast foods and processed foods. You need fiber to regulate your bowels, for good colon health and for weight loss if you are overweight. Eating fruits and vegetables increases your fiber intake. Juicing makes it easy. You might also supplement with psyllium fiber and bran fiber.

How you combine your foods is also important. The best combinations are proteins or fats with vegetables, vegetables with simple carbohydrates or vegetables with fat. Combining your fruit with protein and healthy fats slows sugar/carbohydrate absorption. In fact, make protein the first bite of each meal to slow absorption even more. That means less fat storage, longer lasting energy and fewer food cravings shortly after you eat. And you will easily accomplish that by eating less. In fact, even if you eat unhealthy food from time to time, eating less of it at each meal can be almost as important as eating the right food.

If you add sweeteners to anything, the healthiest sugar substitute we know of is stevia. Stevia is a delicious natural herb sweetener with added health benefits. You can find it your local health food store. Avoid artificial sweeteners. Most are toxic and can undermine your health.

For example, high doses of aspartame may lead to neurodegeneration. Aside from the damage it can do to your brain, aspartame can cause cancer. One well-controlled, peer-reviewed, seven-year study even found that as little as 20 mg per day can cause cancer in humans. One 12-ounce diet soda contains about 180 mg of aspartame, so you do the math for that risk!

It can also lead to multiple sclerosis, Parkinson's disease, Alzheimer's disease, memory and hearing loss and hormonal problems.

How about Splenda? That's harmless, right? Well, look at what a study, published in the *Journal of Toxicology and Environmental Health* found. Splenda reduces the amount of good bacteria in your intestines by 50 percent, contributes to weight gain, increases the pH level in your intestines (bad for your digestion) and affects a glycoprotein in your body that can have crucial health effects, particularly if you're on certain medications.

"Diet soda anyone?"

In addition to changing what you eat, consider changing when you eat. The fluctuations in your insulin levels, which are so damaging to your system, can be controlled by eating smaller, more frequent meals. This will also boost your metabolism, causing calories to be burned faster, and will raise your energy level.

Longevity Express Dietary Recommendations:

➢ Reduce your simple carbohydrate intake by removing refined sugars and starches from your diet. The first things to go should be candy, cookies and soda. Pasta and white breads are also problems and should be eliminated.

➢ Replace the above carbohydrates with at least six servings of brightly-colored fresh or frozen vegetables and one to three servings of fruit each day. One serving equals one-half cup. Fruits and vegetables are nutrient dense sources of carbohydrates and contain loads of essential vitamins and minerals, many of which are terrific antioxidants (to be discussed in Chapter Seven, Nutritional Supplements).

➢ Combine fruit with protein and healthy fats to slow sugar absorption.

➢ Eat lean protein, including protein from organically grown plant foods, spirulina and "broken cell wall" chlorella. Plants have one-seventh the contaminants of most commercial animal products. Eat three servings of quality protein per day, including hempseed or egg white protein powder. One serving equals three ounces of meat.

➢ Be cautious with fried foods. Deep-fried foods and solid fats (butter, margarine and lard) are especially damaging to your digestive and cardiovascular system. If you do eat fried foods, fry with macadamia oil or coconut oil, and stir fry rather than deep fry. Use macadamia oil or coconut oil for all your cooking needs. Both have a high smoking point and are ideal for sautéing and cooking. Macadamia oil tastes almost like butter and has the lowest Omega-6 fatty acids of all cooking oils and the highest monounsaturated fats of all cooking oils. While extra virgin olive oil can, and should be, included in your diet, do not use it to cook with.

It is highly susceptible to oxidative damage when heated. Only add it cold to salads and other dishes.

➢ Replace bad fats with good fats. You need fats to absorb many vitamins and to have cells function properly. Low-fat diets trigger famine response and increased production of body fat. Get most of your fats from monounsaturated fats and essential fatty acids. Saturated fats are found in meat and are not the villains they are accused of being. Trans-fatty acids are the real culprits. They're basically unsaturated oils treated with hydrogen to create an artificial saturated fat. A perfect example is heated French fries. Eat fresh olives, extra virgin olive oil, avocados, seeds and nuts, and supplement with fish oil. Forget flaxseed oil, but freshly ground organic flaxseeds are at the top of my food list.

➢ There is so much information about healthy versus unhealthy fats out there, and I realize it can be confusing. But I can sum up the difference between a healthy fat and an unhealthy one in one word: "natural." If it was made by man, in a lab, as opposed to naturally in a plant or animal, just pass. Just about every naturally occurring fat you can think of is great for your health. This includes the natural fats in animal products. When choosing which dairy products and meats to include in your diet, always keep in mind these tips to live by:

• Dairy products should be raw (unpasteurized) if you absolutely refuse to do without them. Yes, pasteurization does kill bacteria. But it also kills beneficial bacteria, destroys enzymes, lowers or wipes out vitamin content, denatures fragile milk proteins and is associated with allergies and more. What happens to pasteurized and homogenized milk when you leave it on a counter? It turns rancid. But raw milk ferments and turns to a beneficial food such as yogurt. Healthy alternatives to milk are almond milk, especially home-made, organic coconut milk and coconut water as well as hemp milk. My favorite brand is Tempt Hempmilk.

It's creamy, delicious, and the unsweetened versions are sugar-free.

- Look for organic meats from grass-fed or free-range animals from a local source.

- Ideally, eat meat items that support your nutritional type.

➢ Increase your intake of fish. Fish oils are rich in omega-3 fatty acids (the good fat), which aid immune function, cardiovascular health and brain health. As you age, your red blood cells lose their elasticity and become sticky. Fish oil helps keep your red blood cells slippery and elastic. Eat fish at least three times per week. But limit your intake of larger fish found at the top of the food chain such as swordfish, tuna and shark because of the high toxic levels of mercury and other contaminants.

➢ Lower your intake of red meat unless it is extremely lean. Most red meat is high in nitrosamines, a compound that has been directly linked to some forms of cancer. It is also much higher in fat than most other meat. It is a myth that all meat causes cancer. There is probably no correlation between cancer and high protein intake, only commercial red meat and cancer. Lean, skinless organic poultry breast is a good substitute with occasional lean red meat. I prefer ostrich as a red meat choice. Ostrich is tasty and has a fraction of the fat found even in turkey. We recommend wild game or bison as well. Lamb may be much healthier than beef, since it is mostly grass-fed and much lower in hormones, antibiotics and other contaminates and lower in saturated fat. However, lamb has a very high fat content, so limit your consumption. In fact, I believe it is best to limit your consumption of most animal products.

➢ A study showed wild African animals contained 3.9% fat, while commercially bred and fed beef contain 25–35%. Does this give you a clue about fast foods? Researchers say eating too much fast food can cause serious damage to your liver in as little as a week. Instead, opt for hempseed protein, egg white protein, whey protein (if you eat dairy), egg whites and beans/legumes (if you eat legumes) as your good protein sources.

➢ Avoid blackened or burnt foods. Food charred to a crisp contains many toxic chemicals and has been implicated in some forms of cancer. It also accelerates glycation. A good rule of thumb is to cook with as low temperatures as possible.

➢ The average person should eat fewer than 2,000 calories a day, or around 12 calories per pound of your optimal weight or 80% of your optimal weight if you're on a caloric-restricted diet.

➢ Your particular metabolic type might determine that you function better with less protein and more carbohydrates or more protein and less carbohydrates. Or more fats, etc. I used to go slightly higher in protein and a little lower in carbohydrates, but then I found out I was a "mixed" metabolic type, which suggested I function better with slightly more complex carbohydrates and slightly less protein.

Another reason I cut back slightly on protein is studies suggest a high protein diet may increase your IGF-1 level, which could possibly shorten your life and increase your cancer risk. This may be attributed to the fact that methionine, one of the body's essential amino acids, is prone to rapid oxidation. That may be a reason to consider increasing your intake of antioxidants if you are on a higher than normal protein diet. Generally, animal protein has much more methionine than plant protein sources. High protein diets can also deplete calcium. But other studies show how lean protein foods drastically reduce your chances of cancer and heart disease. The common 40:40:20 ratio will shift toward more complex carbohydrates (fruits and vegetables) if you are observing a strict reduced calorie diet. I have adopted a Paleo diet which calls for a ratio of roughly 33:30:37 including high omega-3 fats. Others suggest 25:25:50 to 20:20:60, with 50-60% of your calories coming from healthy fats.

➢ Graze, or eat smaller meals that are less spaced out throughout the day. Five to six smaller meals are much healthier than three large meals. Even though you might eat the same number of calories as you would with three meals a day, grazers won't gain the weight. Grazing also keeps your energy high, your body strong and your mind alert while improving your digestion, nutrient absorption and metabolism. Maybe make one or two of your meals a highly nutritious and well-balanced energy shake or green smoothie.

➢ Drink plenty of filtered water (at least one-half ounce a day for each pound of body weight), eliminate soda, and reduce coffee from your diet. (Recent studies have shown coffee consumption can dramatically reduce the risk of stroke, heart disease, diabetes, cancer, liver disease, cognitive decline and DNA damage. However, you can get similar benefits from supplementing with chlorogenic acid, a polyphenol found in the green coffee bean. Polyphenols are potent antioxidant compounds in plant foods.)

➢ Inflammation and glycation damage your immune system and promote disease as seen in Chapter Three. So, stay away from refined foods. Low-fat varieties are usually high in sugar. Whole grain foods, if you choose to eat them, and fresh fruit have more fiber and are converted to sugars more gradually. Fiber also prevents carcinogens from entering your bloodstream. To control inflammation, lower your blood sugar level, lose weight, exercise more, reduce stress, avoid or cut back on red meat and alcohol. Limit egg yolks to six a week, and take a daily baby or whole aspirin with your biggest meal under a doctor's supervision.

➤ Reduce your intake of commercial dairy products in particular, or eliminate all dairy in general. Commercial cow's milk has up to 59 active hormones, scores of allergens, fat and cholesterol, and much of it contains herbicides, pesticides, dioxins and up to 52 powerful antibiotics. Get your calcium from non-dairy sources. You'll find calcium in every natural food we eat. For example, a cup of sesame seeds contains ten times the calcium as a cup of milk.

➤ Add spices to your diet. Many contain powerful antioxidants, and they can do wonders for taste. Some of the better ones are cayenne, garlic, turmeric, cumin, rosemary, oregano and paprika.

➤ Eat a balanced breakfast to help you lose weight, increase your strength, boost your brainpower and focus, lower your stress and decrease fat storage. Of people who lost an average of seventy pounds and kept it off for six years, only 4% said they ever skipped breakfast.

➤ Reduce your consumption of foods that require labels.

➤ Introduce probiotics into your diet. (See the next section on Digestion). The *Bacillus Coagulans* strain is good. Its main benefits are it survives the acidic environment of your stomach, making it to your small intestine where it does the most good, and it does not need to be refrigerated. Infintis, Reuteri, Ultimate Flora Critical Care 50 Billion and Dura Flora are also excellent. They are therapeutic to the colon and strengthen colon health.

➤ I also suggest prebiotics such as FOS (FructoOligoSaccharides). They are used by the beneficial bacteria in your colon as a food source, promoting the growth of beneficial bacteria, which suppress harmful organisms.

You could keep it simple by adopting the Mediterranean diet. Italians and people in Southern France stack up well against strict vegetarians when it comes to health statistics. (Most vegetarians do not eat many vegetables. They load up on grains which tend to make them very unhealthy.) The Mediterranean diet emphasizes fresh fruits and veggies, whole grains, garlic, olive oil, tomatoes and tomato sauce, moderate amounts of fish and poultry, some lean red meat—and one glass of red wine a day. Although it's low in saturated fats, perhaps the most significant thing about the Mediterranean style diet is the absence of processed foods, which are loaded with sugars and dangerous trans fats.

If you think you can't carve out enough of your time to master these guidelines, why not put a good nutritionist on your team? You might contact Prof. Joe Carrington at carrington@post.harvard.edu.

Apples or Bananas for Longevity?

How do you really know what to eat? What foods are best for longevity, for your heart, for losing or gaining weight, to reverse or avoid type 2 diabetes and for your overall health in general?

How about all the words and terms thrown at you like nutrient density, enzymes, ATP, BMI? How do you determine what they mean without doing an individual search on each one? And how do they relate to or interact with one another? What impact do they have on you... which ones are more important for you and which don't apply to your particular situation?

Do you really know the differences between different types of fiber, how much you need and why... and the best way to get them?

Inflammation is a life-shortener and a major contributor to virtually every disease. While inflammation is an epidemic of extreme proportions, there's no reason for most of us to be inflamed. Which foods are the best inflammation fighters?

We know how bad fast foods are for us, yet many of us still eat them. Sometimes it's just, well, convenient. And it's hard to beat them for taste, isn't it? Wouldn't it be nice to know which are best for you?

And wouldn't it be cool to have a simple quick way to track the nutrients, calories and more in everything you eat, any day you want? And finally, you can be one click away from knowing exactly what foods best suit your particular needs.

Ya gotta love the Internet, because there's a website that gives you all the above and waaay more. This is one you should bookmark for sure. It's for the casual user as well as for the serious food researcher. I just love this site: www.nutritiondata.self.com

Acid/Alkaline Balance

Acid and alkaline refer to the acid base characteristics of any liquid.

Your health is extremely sensitive to the tiniest change in your pH levels. We often hear about how acidosis, or being too acidic, can lead to disease. Cancer cells thrive in a highly acidic environment. Alkalosis, or being too alkaline, is much rarer and can cause problems as well. Ideally, the relative pH of your blood balance should be around 7.4. The lower you go on the scale, the more acidic, and the higher, the more alkaline. A balance of 7.0 is perfectly neutral, so 7.4 is slightly alkaline.

Many people call certain foods "acidic" and others "alkaline." This is a little misleading. Measuring the pH of food outside your body is irrelevant. How your food is metabolized is what happens to it after it is digested and absorbed. After most of the components of food are oxidized, you have minerals left over that are alkaline, acidic or neutral. The minerals that are found in fruits and vegetables are alkaline forming and lead to good health and a strong immune system.

The minerals found in proteins, mostly in meat, fish, poultry, eggs, cheese, grains, legumes, most nuts and salt are acid forming. Salt is especially toxic. Because of its high chloride content, salt is one of the worst offenders in making your diet acidic. Other foods that don't contain protein such as soft drinks and coffee are extremely acid forming.

According to William Wolcott, although red meat is generally considered to be acidic, it can be alkalinic for pure strong protein types, while fruits and some veggies make them acidic. William Wolcott is a recognized metabolic typing authority. It pays to know your metabolic type.

Except for salt, soft drinks and coffee (and cheese, grains and legumes if you follow a hunter-gatherer diet) your body needs a balance of alkaline and acid forming foods. So just because a food is acid forming doesn't necessarily mean it is bad for you.

But most of us are too acidic. To avoid colds and flu and other more serious disorders, keep your body slightly alkaline.

You will normally need a large amount of vegetables and fruits to optimize your body's pH acid/alkaline balance, so you might supplement with the four alkaline minerals; calcium, magnesium, potassium and sodium. You might even try a teaspoon of baking soda in a large glass of water. This will cost you pennies.

How else can you alkalinize your body? Exercise and deep breathing. We cover those in Chapters Six and Ten.

Digestion

Let's wind down our diet chapter with a few words on digestion.

Most people don't realize that about 70% of your immune system is located in your digestive system. That means a healthy gut is your major focal point, since you want to maintain optimal health. Remember, a robust immune system is your number one defense system against all disease.

Undigested food doesn't magically disappear. It passes into the colon where it is fermented by intestinal bacteria. Then a related reaction called putrefaction emits a long list of toxins. As you know, indigestion can be awfully uncomfortable. How often did you feel bloated after a meal or get gas or abdominal pain? Here are six easy steps to improve your digestion:

1. Again, graze. Eat small amounts spread over four to six meals a day instead of stuffing yourself two to three times a day.

2. Chew your food well.

3. Eat slowly. The heaviest people tend to eat fast. Since it takes about twenty minutes for your brain to recognize you are full, the faster you eat, the more you overeat. Think of your meal as a series of first bites. You'll savor your food, improve your digestion and eat less. Eating slowly also tends to lower your blood glucose levels. Take small bites over a long period of time, and chew each mouthful of food at least twenty to thirty times. If your biggest meal takes you less than thirty minutes, you are probably eating too fast.

4. Don't wash your food down with a beverage. Chew well, swallow and then take a sip of room temperature water, tea or maybe red wine. Stay away from ice cold beverages with your meals.

5. Relax while you eat.

6. Supplement with a high quality probiotic, a supplement containing friendly bacteria. Without good gut bacteria, your body can't absorb certain undigested starches and sugars. And it doesn't absorb minerals and break down toxins efficiently. Normally, you don't need to take probiotics forever, but they can be incredibly helpful when you eat excess grains or sugar, or if you have to take antibiotics. Taking a high-quality probiotic for a month, every 30–60 days, will typically help your digestive system function efficiently.

    You may not need probiotic supplements, though. Cultured foods like yogurt and sauerkraut are good sources of natural, healthy bacteria. And fermented foods, such as natto, can give your body the similar benefits of consuming a whole bottle of good bacteria, at a fraction of the cost.

As you can see, you can follow our guidelines and still enjoy eating. In fact, if you like to eat, you should have extra incentive to live longer. Just think—if you add only five years to your life—that means you get to eat at least 5,500 more meals.

Top Ten Foods for Longer Life

They're all backed by major independent studies.

1. Tomatoes: Tomatoes contain a very powerful antioxidant called lycopene. Studies show lycopene cuts cancer rates by 40% and heart disease by 50%. And it makes the elderly function better mentally. Tomato sauce has five times as much lycopene as fresh tomatoes. And surprisingly, jarred tomatoes have three times as much.

2. Olive oil: Reduces death from heart disease and cancer. Use extra virgin olive oil.

3. Red or purple grapes: Grape juice and red wine increase longevity. Two alcoholic drinks per day maximum.

4. Garlic: Packed with antioxidants. It fights cancer and heart disease and overall is anti-aging.

5. Spinach: Follows right behind garlic for antioxidant protection. It's rich in folic acid, which helps fight cancer, heart disease and mental disorders and may help prevent Alzheimer's. According to a featured study in the *Journal of Nutritional Biochemistry*, plasma concentrations of the B vitamin folate (folic acid) correspond to telomere length in both men and women via its maintenance of DNA integrity and DNA methylation.

6. Salmon and other fatty fish: These contain lots of omega-3 fatty acids, which fight virtually every disease and keep your brain and heart functioning optimally. They also lower inflammation. Caution: make sure your salmon is wild Pacific or Alaskan salmon. Farm and Atlantic salmon can be contaminated.

7. Nuts: Eat over five ounces per week. They can cut heart attack deaths by 40% in women. People who eat about two ounces of nuts four times a week tend to live up to two to three years longer! A large-scale, 30-year long study found that people who regularly ate one ounce of nuts at least seven times per

week were 20 percent less likely to die for any reason (New England Journal of Medicine November 21, 2013). Almonds and walnuts lower cholesterol. Unsalted are best for you. And eat them raw if you can. You may want to avoid nuts altogether during pregnancy if you have a family history of asthma. If you have most any disease, or any kind of insulin-related problems, you may want to avoid large amounts of seeds and nuts except for flax, chia and walnuts.

8. Blueberries: High in antioxidants. One-half cup a day can retard aging and block brain changes leading to fading memory. Other dark, richly colored berries run neck-and-neck with blueberries.

9. Matcha green tea and black tea (maybe white too): One cup per day can cut heart disease risk in half. (Note: Instant or bottled have little effect) Other beneficial effects include improved mental alertness; lower blood cholesterol and triglyceride levels; reduced blood pressure; lower risk of breast, colon, lung, ovarian and prostate cancers; protection against type 2 diabetes; improved exercise performance and lowered risk of obesity.

10. Pomegranate: New studies show pomegranate to be one of the richer sources of antioxidants. More about pomegranate later.

Fasting

How about fasting? There are pros and cons about extended fasts, but nearly everyone agrees that skipping meals or fasting gives your digestive system a rest and helps detoxify your system if your diet is unhealthy. If you are a carbohydrate nutritional type who fares better with a high complex carbohydrate diet, you might do better with fasting than a protein nutritional type who functions better with a lot of protein.

Fasting helps, because what you eat, drink and breathe all have the potential to increase your toxic load. Ditto for what you put on your skin. Even though your lungs, liver, kidneys and your skin are designed to remove your toxins, they are stretched beyond their limits in today's polluted world. So it's up to you to periodically cleanse your system if you want to keep toxins from prematurely aging you and making you sick. You can do this by either periodically fasting or detoxifying. You might consider both.

Fasting is simple and easy. I recommend short fasts, two to four days every month. Or you might try two days every two weeks or one day every week. I fast one day a week—no food for 24 hours.

If you abstain from food completely, drink only filtered water or distilled water and bone broth. For even better results, you might drink two to three large mugs of hot filtered water each fast day with two tablespoons of raw apple cider vinegar and one teaspoon of raw honey.

You can get the beneficial effects of caloric restriction (CR) if you eat as much as you want every other day and fast every other day. Besides being the only proven way to extend maximum lifespans in mammals, CR is also an effective way to dodge diabetes, heart disease and nearly every other disease associated with aging.

Another form of fasting is going on a CR 7 eating schedule. This means you utilize a concept called "intermittent fasting" (IF) to redistribute and lose body fat and to simulate CR. Do not eat past 6 PM, and do not eat before 11 AM. By doing so, you go on a 17 hour fast every day. According to a 2005 article in Lancet, mice and rats maintained on an intermittent fasting regimen lived up to 30% longer than those fed otherwise.

On IF, the longest time you'll ever abstain from food is 36 hours, although 14-18 hours is more common. Skipping breakfast is far easier and logistically and socially more acceptable, but avoiding dinner might be better from a health perspective.

Our genes are optimized for this type of feeding schedule. It takes about six to eight hours for your body to metabolize your glycogen stores, and after that, you actually start to shift to burning fat. However, if you are replenishing your glycogen by eating every few hours, you make it far more difficult for your body to actually use your fat stores as fuel.

Surprisingly, hunger is not the problem you might think. Fasting also has a profound effect on your food cravings. It shifts cravings toward more subtle tasting, nutrient dense, satiety-pro-moting foods, which can then lead to a spontaneous decrease in your overall calorie intake.

When following an IF regimen, make your diet low glyce-mic and high in protein and fiber. Eat whole foods, along with nutrient dense antioxidant foods. Don't even think about IF if you eat the typical American portions of high glycemic junk food.

Importantly, our ancestors did not eat regular meals like we do today. They ate when they killed or found food and when they had some stored food left over. Extended periods between meals were normal. Our bodies are still programmed to miss meals. That's one reason you should break up your regular meal schedule or grazing with some type of intermittent fasting.

Is IF as effective as CR? More research will tell, but its benefits are profound.

More Fasting Benefits

Could fasting for two days a week prevent age-related brain shrinkage, heart disease, diabetes, and possibly even cancer? New research suggests that fasting triggers a variety of health-promot-ing hormonal and metabolic changes.

Fasting has been shown to reduce:

- Bad" LDL cholesterol

- Total cholesterol

- Triglycerides

- Inflammation levels

- Free radical damage

Fasting also normalizes your insulin sensitivity, which is key for optimal health. Insulin resistance (which is what you get when your insulin sensitivity plummets) is a primary contributing factor to nearly all chronic disease, from diabetes to heart disease and even cancer.

Except for intermittent fasting, fasting usually does, but does not necessarily mean abstaining from ALL food, but rather a dramatic reduction of caloric intake. You should cut your daily calories at least in half, and preferably consume no more than 500-800 calories a day during your fasts. That's not so tough, is it?

"Suddenly dropping your food intake <u>dramatically</u>, cutting it by at least half for a <u>day</u> or so, triggers protective processes in the brain," explains Professor Mark Mattson, head of neuroscience at the U.S. National <u>Institute</u> on Aging.

He adds, "It is similar to the beneficial effect you get from exercise."

Hunger seems to benefit your physical shape and longevity similarly to physical exercise. When manipulated properly, hunger has shown to trigger mechanisms that increase your energy, repair your tissues and keep you in prime physical shape.

Interestingly, some of the mechanisms largely responsible for weight loss and diabetic control when fasting are also the ones responsible for the benefits to your brain. Research suggests that caloric restriction can protect brain cells and make them more resilient against stress. This protective effect is partly due to fasting's effect on leptin and ghrelin; two hormones involved in appetite regulation. According to Professor Mattson, these hormones are also involved in the process of renewing brain cells—especially in the hippocampus—*when you are not overweight.*

This could help protect your brain against memory loss and degenerative diseases such as Alzheimer's and Parkinson's.

How Fasting Triggers Your Longevity Genes

Your body thrives when under nutritional and physical stress. Both caloric restriction and physical hardship are perceived by your body as survival signals to adapt and improve.

The effects of caloric restriction and physical hardship on longevity seem to be deeply rooted in your biology. Both trigger biological mechanisms that evolved to help humans endure times of food scarcity and extreme physical hardship. When triggered, these mechanisms compensate your body by protecting your insulin system, strengthening your immune defenses, improving your tissue restoration and upgrading your muscle fiber quality.

To trigger your longevity genes, you need to routinely challenge your body. You need to train and feed your body as it's originally designed to operate.

It has been widely agreed that the human body is not programmed for a world of plenty. Your body declines and deteriorates by chronic indulgence and lack of challenge.

It's starting to look like the longevity benefits of fasting can be attributed to the degree of caloric restriction. That is, fasting is total caloric restriction, while CR is partial. When you fast, you're going whole hog. You're subjecting yourself to an acute stressor, getting the hormetic benefits, and then recovering from that stressor by eating normally thereafter (until you do it again). When you calorie restrict, you're undergoing a chronic stressor. Day in, day out, you're worrying about food, restricting energy and nutrient intake, and there's really no period of recovery. You're always residing in a partially restricted state, drifting from paltry meal to paltry meal. There is no feast.

There's one more advantage of intermittent fasting over CR. We now know that it appears to conserve more lean mass than CR.

Fasting and Exercise: Are They Compatible?

Fasting affects your muscles similar to physical exercise. Besides stabilizing your insulin and accelerating fat burning, fasting activates genes and growth factors which regenerate new brain and muscle cells.

In the brain, fasting promotes activation of stem cells, making them committed to restore and regenerate new neurons. In the muscle, fasting turns on satellite cells to commit, differentiate and fuse into new muscle cells.

Fasting is the most powerful trigger of muscle tissue recycling. It increases removal of broken proteins and damaged cells to allow synthesis of new protein and regeneration of new muscle cells for repair and sustainability.

So periodic (intermittent) fasting may prove to be a most effective anti-aging strategy as well as a key weight loss tool… and even more so, when combined with exercise.

For muscle rejuvenation, you need to initiate muscle catabolism to remove and recycle broken proteins and damaged cells. This can be done by increasing the gap between your meals and exercising while fasting. This regimen seems to be most effective in activating mechanisms that repair and rejuvenate your tissues.

For muscle buildup on the other hand, you need to promote muscle anabolism. You can achieve that by feeding your muscles with frequent, fast assimilating protein meals throughout the day including 2-3 post exercise recovery meals. This pulse feeding regimen has shown to yield maximum protein utilization efficiency.

Fitness expert Ori Hofmekler also concluded fasting has the surprising benefit of helping you reconstruct your muscles when combined with exercise. This is due to an ingenious preservation mechanism that protects your active muscles from wasting. In a nutshell, if you don't have sufficient fuel in your system when you exercise, your body will break down other tissues *but not the active muscle*, i.e. the muscle being exercised.

Cutting down on your grains and sugars, replacing them with high quality fats and skipping some meals, especially before exercise, seem to be a powerful combination to help you take control of your well-being.

Detoxifying

If you're average, you may be carrying around pounds of putrefying sludge in your colon. Get rid of it. It is aging you before your time by reducing your body's ability to absorb nutrients. It also makes you sick by dumping its rotting by-products into your system.

A pure diet coupled with regular exercise is your best way to remove toxins from your body and to keep them from accumulating in the first place. Some people recommend a three-week purification program every three months as well as annual full body cleansing. For detailed information on detoxifying your body, you might get a copy of *Detoxify or Die* by Dr. Sherry A. Rogers. If you decide to buy any detox, cleansing or purification products, make sure companies selling them can back up their claims with hard data.

The "Healthiest" Alcoholic Beverages

To drink or not to drink? What's the purpose of living longer if you can't enjoy yourself? We're not encouraging drinking. Just limit yourself to two drinks a day if you do drink. And that doesn't mean not drinking at all six days a week and having fourteen on the seventh. Drink sensibly. Besides social issues, drinking more than one or two a day for the average sized person can wreak havoc on your body and lead to all kinds of long-term physical and mental problems.

If you decide to imbibe, remember, alcohol is a toxin. Drinking too much on a regular basis has been linked to weight gain, high blood pressure, stroke, heart disease, dementia, osteoporosis, certain cancers and dry wrinkled skin.

If you drink, we suggest eating before or during drinking, and drinking water with your alcoholic beverages. We recommend only beverages made without grains such as the following:

Red wine. Dry wines have less sugar. In general, most red wines have little or no sugar. Most sweet wines are white. A four ounce glass of dry red wine usually contains about 83 calories, no sugar, .5 grams of carbohydrates and no fat. Many people claim health benefits for moderate red wine consumption.

Tequila. One shot contains around 97 calories, no fat and no carbs as well as no sugar. There is even a bit of potassium.

Brandy. Unflavored brandy has about 72 calories per shot, no sugar and zero fat and carbs. The sugar has been removed in the distillation process.

Rum. The unflavored versions have about 64 calories per shot. They also contain no sugar, fat or carbs.

Bottoms up if you must, but not too often.

So in summing up our diet chapter, be aware of the consequences of over-drinking, overeating and of an unhealthy diet. With the way science is charging forward, you may be eating and drinking yourself into missing the super-longevity train.

You will live a long, healthy life to the extent you can: prevent oxidation; reduce inflammation; prevent glycation; and enhance methylation. Start with your diet. Climb aboard the Express today. You'll never have a chance to relive this moment.

As new nutritional strategies are discovered, we can notify you. Simply visit www.MaxLife.org/sssbook now in order to be alerted.

Now on to your second biggest life extender.

CHAPTER 6. STEP 2—EXERCISE

"There is no drug in current or prospective use that holds as much promise for sustained health as a lifetime program of physical exercise."

—*Journal of the American Medical Association*

If Exercise Were a Drug, It Would Dominate the Headlines

There was a time when physicians advised people to take it easy as they grew older. It has now been definitively shown that lack of activity at any age will torpedo your health. People who are inactive show many signs of accelerated aging including: bone loss, poor cardiovascular tone, decreased telomere length and increased incidence of heart disease, cancer and diabetes as compared to physically active people. And according to one study, the odds of developing Alzheimer's were nearly quadrupled in people who were less active during their leisure time between the ages of twenty and sixty, compared with their more active peers.

Other studies suggest more than 400,000 Americans die each year from poor diet and inactivity. That accounts for 17% of all deaths! Only tobacco accounts for more fatalities, and just barely.

Also, research shows your muscle mass is the major factor in your longevity and in your quality of life. Recently, doctors in England compared the waist circumferences, biceps masses, and body mass indexes of 4,107 men ages sixty to seventy-nine. They found that men with both above average biceps and smaller than average waists were 64% less likely to die within six years than other men in the study.

Exercise reduces disease and death dramatically for *all* major progressive diseases. According to a study involving over 13,000 participants cited by Ray Kurzweil in *The Future of Aging*, the overall death rate for moderate exercisers was 60% less than the sedentary group—and the high fitness group scored much better. Yet some 70% of Americans do not participate in any type of physical activity.

Even Brief Exercise Gives More Life, Produces Genetic Changes and Treats Disease

Those 70% should read the August 17, 2011 issue of *The Herald*. It cited a study from the Institute of Population Science at the National Health Research Institutes in Zhunan, Taiwan published in *The Lancet*. That study found as little as 15 minutes of physical activity a day can reduce the risk of dying by 14% and increase lifespan by three years.

More exercise led to more life gains. Every additional 15 minutes of daily exercise further reduced all-cause death rates by 4%. This trend continued until a person was exercising for 100 minutes a day, after which no further benefit was seen.

More vigorous activity for shorter periods of time had the same effect as less intense exercise carried out for longer. After every session of intense exercise, you grow a little stronger, more alert, energetic and joyful.

Research published in the journal *Cell Metabolism* shows that when healthy but inactive people exercise intensely, even if the exercise is brief, it produces an immediate positive change in their DNA. A genetic activation increases the production of fat-busting proteins and compounds that help stabilize your blood sugar.

Normalizing your glucose and insulin levels by optimizing insulin receptor sensitivity is perhaps *the most important factor for optimizing your overall health and preventing chronic disease.* At some research centers, participants were able to improve their insulin sensitivity an average of 24 percent with as little as three minutes of high intensity training (HIT) per week. (More on HIT later in this chapter).

Exercise can also treat serious diseases such as cancer. A new report issued by Macmillan Cancer Support argues that exercise should be part of standard cancer care. It recommends that all patients getting cancer treatment should be told to engage in moderate-intensity exercise for two and a half hours every week.

A previous study by Harvard Medical School researchers found that breast cancer patients who exercise moderately for three to five hours a week cut their odds of dying from cancer by about half. In fact, *any amount* of weekly exercise increased a patient's odds of surviving breast cancer. This benefit also remained constant regardless of whether women were diagnosed early on or after their cancer had spread. Finally, research has found that exercise reduces the risk of breast cancer recurrence by about 40%.

Research has also shown that exercise can reduce your risk of dying from prostate cancer by up to 30%.

Remember that even if you're chronically ill, exercise can be a potent ally. That said, if you have cancer or any other chronic disease, you will of course need to tailor your exercise routine to your individual scenario, taking into account your stamina and current health. For example, you may at times need to exercise at a lower intensity, or for shorter durations. But do make a concerted effort to keep yourself moving. As mentioned above, even cancer patients should aim for *a minimum* of 2.5 hours of exercise a week, at moderate intensity, to boost their chances of successful recovery.

Always listen to your body, and if you feel you need a break, take time to rest. But even exercising for just a few minutes a day is better than not exercising at all.

Exercise is critical to help dodge or reduce diabetes as well as most other diseases. According to the American Diabetes Association, exercising moderately for only thirty minutes a day coupled with a 5–10% reduction in body weight resulted in an astonishing 58% reduction in diabetes. They also report that 90% of all people with diabetes are overweight.

Any exercise that gets the heart pumping may even reduce the risk of dementia and slow the condition's progression once it starts, reported a Mayo Clinic study published in the September 2011 issue of *Mayo Clinic Proceedings.*

Eric Ahlskog, M.D., Ph.D., a neurologist at Mayo Clinic said: "We concluded that you can make a very compelling argument for exercise as a disease-modifying strategy to prevent dementia and mild cognitive impairment, and for favorably modifying these processes once they have developed."

You Either Grow or Regress, Nothing Stands Still

Your cells constantly turn over. You are either growing or decaying. In fact, life's a cycle of growth and decay. Exercise is the master signaler to make growth outbalance decay. Lethargy accelerates decay and suppresses growth.

Exercise and mood share the same chemistry. Lifestyle and exercise signals send billions of growth messages to and from your brain to make you smarter, stronger and sexier, even with advancing age. So instead of considering it as exercise, think of it as food for growth, agility, independence, looks and youthfulness.

It naturally follows that people who feel better perform better. Why do you think many companies are installing gyms for their employees?

Sure, exercise is tiring for 30-60 minutes if done properly. But then it energizes you the rest of the time. Inactivity may feel good at first, but it makes you tired all day, every day. Activity is in tune with nature. It promotes growth. Inactivity is counter to nature. It decays you. So you can be lazy and tired and simply surviving—or active and energetic and alive. It's your choice.

And the best news? It takes much less effort to keep your gains than it did to achieve them. The brain can't always accept that, but it's the truth!

Your biochemistry responds negatively to overeating and being sedentary. Idleness signals the decay. Evolution designed you to be active. Don't be fooled by your air conditioned SUV. Genetically speaking, you are still a caveman—hard-wired to move seven days a week and to be fit enough to cope with your environment. Abundance and idleness are foreign to your genome. No matter what you think of exercise, you were still designed to hunt. It's embedded in your genome. Act counter to your genetic makeup, and you will decay. Act in harmony with it, and you will thrive.

The problem is, our bodies don't know how to read our biggest killer—this new abundance. We lie around and eat ourselves to death. Your mind is not programmed for idleness. It's programmed to be alert to danger and to hunt and to gather.

But civilization, from the evolutionary standpoint, rapidly changed our lifestyle. So now we're suddenly soft, and our bodies rebel. The only reason we live longer is because of modern medicine, less environmental risk factors and low risks of famine. At the end though, we suffer from diseases our ancestors never had—diseases you can mostly avoid.

But you don't have to hunt and gather. Exercise can be fun. Your biochemistry only recognizes your activity. To keep it fun and interesting, and to maximize your results, do a variety of different exercises and intensities and cross-train. And when activity is fun, it becomes addictive. Besides, it's simply not an option if you want to be independent, well, pain-free, energetic and good looking.

So train like a caveman. That's how you are designed. Why fight nature? Emulate hunting and gathering. Hunting was essentially high intensity interval training (HIIT). It builds muscle and alertness. Do HIIT 2-3 days a week. Gathering simulated activity, or long, slow exercise, burns fat and builds endurance. This could be anything that has you breathing hard while still being able to carry on a conversation for 45 minutes or so.

If you're at 60-65% of your maximum heart rate, you're in a good zone. This best life extending range may be vigorous exercise, but not exhausting for most of your training sessions. Make sure you break a sweat and breathe hard. If not, you're missing the biggest benefits.

Mother Nature programmed us to survive if we are fit and to exit the gene pool if we're not. Exercise was the primary difference among those studied, but your diet and supplements contribute to your muscle mass, too.

By the way, youngsters can get away with lack of exercise more than adults. When you are young, your body is forgiving, and it can take a little abuse. But we need exercise more as we get older, because we start to break down. Some think the older you get, the harder it is to exercise. It really isn't though, and the rewards are over the top.

Other than some key stem cells in each organ or your brain cells, your trillions of cells live for a few weeks or months on average, depending on each cell type. Then they die and are replaced by new cells. Your whole body is practically replaced every three months. Only you choose whether that "new" body is stronger or weaker—younger or older.

It's Never Too Late

Despite your body beginning to wear out as you age, there is still much you can do to slow and reverse the trend. As part of a long-term study to determine how post-middle age changes in physical activity affect mortality rates, 2,205 Swedish men were initially surveyed from 1970 to 1973 at the age of 50. Each participant was categorized into one of four groups according to their level of physical activity: sedentary, low, medium or high. Researchers followed up as they turned 60, 70, 77 and 82.

The study team found what you would expect: exercising more translated into lower mortality rates in all exercising groups. But the study also revealed some surprising findings. Those who raised their level of physical activity between the ages of 50 and 60 experienced the same mortality rates as those men who had always maintained high levels of physical activity.

The results were so pronounced that the study team compared the reduction in mortality to people who stop smoking. "Increased physical activity in middle age is eventually followed by a reduction in mortality to the same level as seen among men with constantly high physical activity. This reduction is comparable with that associated with smoking cessation," writes the study team. However, the researchers found that in order for low-level exercisers to "catch up," they would need to maintain regular physical activity for at least five years.

The study was published in the British Medical Journal. It confirms we can reverse some of the damage done in earlier years and become as healthy as people who have maintained a healthy life-style for most of their lives. In fact, researchers at the University of Pittsburgh finally answered the question, "Is physical frailty inevitable as we grow older?" That question preoccupies scientists and the middle-aged. Until recently, the evidence was disheartening.

A large number of studies in the past few years showed that after age 40, people typically lose 8 percent or more of their muscle mass each decade. Then the process accelerates significantly after age 70. Less muscle mass generally means less strength, mobility and independence. It also has been linked with premature mortality. But a growing body of newer science suggests that such decline may not be inexorable. A study published in the October, 2011 issue of *The Physician and Sportsmedicine* gives us new hope.

The new thinking goes like this: Exercise and you might be able to rewrite the future for your muscles. Researchers found there was little evidence of deterioration in the older athletes' musculature. The athletes in their 70s and 80s had almost as much thigh muscle mass as the athletes in their 40s, with minor, if any fat infiltration. The athletes also remained strong. There was a drop-off in leg muscle strength around age 60 in both men and women. They weren't as strong as the 50-year-olds, but the differential was not huge, and little additional decline followed.

That means the 70 and 80-year-old athletes were about as strong as those in their 60s. So people don't have to lose muscle mass and function as they grow older. The changes that we've assumed were due to aging, and therefore unstoppable, seem actually to be caused by inactivity. And that can be changed.

So Start Moving Now

You are designed to move. When you exercise, your body signals your cells to grow. These growth signals cause a ripple effect, spreading the growth process to every cell in your body, making you functionally younger. Sedentary muscles trickle chemicals, signalling every cell to wither away. It's simple. You can spend the rest of your life in a powerful healthy body, or you can opt for the lazy way to decay. It's your choice, and by riding the Express, you choose health and power.

Sedentary people who get fit cut their heart attack risk by 75–80% over five years. That's impressive, since heart disease is our single biggest killer. According to the *Harvard Alumni Health Study,* you need vigorous activity to significantly lower your risk from coronary heart disease.

Many people in their sixties, seventies and older exercise their way to being in better shape than the average thirty-five-year-old. If you're not exercising now, you can double your strength in three months and maybe double it again in three more months. It doesn't matter if you're twenty-five or eighty-five. In fact, muscle growth in the elderly was statistically equivalent to youngsters doing the same amount of training.

So you're never too old to add strength and flexibility. Researchers also found that percentage of body fat and aerobic capacity was related more to training than to age.

Regular exercise also seems to maintain the levels of hormones that typically decline with age. This is great for your appearance, attitude and your sex drive. (Did you know sex sends longevity signals to your cells that may postpone senescence and death?) Regular exercise helps to increase DHEA and reduce cortisol, the stress hormone. Some of the other general effects of exercise include increased metabolism and increased lymph flow.

One concern over exercise used to be that it produces bursts of free radicals. This is due to the increased use of oxygen by cells in the body in response to greater exertion. As your metabolic rate goes up, you produce greater amounts of free radicals.

In the short-term this has been shown to be detrimental. But in the long-term, people who practice a regular exercise routine for twenty minutes or more three to seven times per week, have a much greater capacity to eliminate free radicals than someone who does not exercise regularly. This greater ability to handle oxidative stress extends to all other potential free radical producing activities; disease, stress, dietary and environmentally source of free radicals. If you'd like to protect yourself from increasing free radicals during exercise, take antioxidants before working out.

If you are over forty years of age, have a chronic disease or any of the following conditions below, check with a doctor before beginning your exercise program.

➢ any new, undiagnosed symptom

➢ chest pain

➢ irregular, rapid or fluttery heart beat

➢ severe shortness of breath

➢ significant, ongoing weight loss that hasn't been diagnosed

➢ infections, such as pneumonia, accompanied by fever

➢ fever itself, which can cause dehydration and a rapid heart beat

➢ acute deep-vein thrombosis (blood clot)

➢ a hernia that is causing symptoms

➢ foot or ankle sores that won't heal

➢ joint swelling

➢ persistent pain or a disturbance in walking after you have fallen (you might have a fracture and not know it, and exercise could cause further injury)

➢ certain eye conditions, such as bleeding in the retina or detached retina (before you exercise after a cataract or lens implant, or after laser treatment or other eye surgery, check with your physician)

➢ artificial joints

You may consider getting a personal fitness trainer to tailor an exercise program for your specific needs and to keep you motivated and on track. Hire a knowledgeable trainer for at least your first few sessions and periodic tune-ups. He or she will guide you into easing into training if you are not in shape. Training builds muscles quickly, but joints take more time to become strong enough to support your stronger muscles.

The best way to stay on track is to decide what kind of activities or sports you enjoy most. Then mimic the basic movements pertaining to those activities, and incorporate those into your routine. Not only will you enjoy training more, but your sports performance should improve as well. Weight training wakes up your neural connections too. This is one reason it improves your performance in your favorite sports. Not only are you stronger and more agile… but you become better coordinated.

Exercise can be generally categorized as either strength training (anaerobic training) or cardio training (aerobic).

Strength Training

Aging cripples us through bone and muscle cell loss, ligaments and tendons drying out and neural degeneration. Strength training prevents and even reverses much of that damage and avoids the suffering that results from the damage. Simply put, weight training makes you look and feel good.

In addition to giving you a greater ability to handle oxidative stress, exercise has very positive effects on your bone density and tendon, ligament, and joint strength. Resistance training (weightlifting) has been shown to have dramatic effects in preventing osteoporosis and connective tissue damage in both men and women of all ages. This effect is enhanced by hormone supplementation in men and especially in women who experience a faster rate of hormonal decline than men. (See Chapter Eight, Anti-Aging Medicine.)

Strength training is the most effective way of slowing down and even reversing the aging process, claim William J. Evans and Irwin H. Rosenburg in their book *Biomarkers*. They cover ten key physiological measures of the aging process and go on to say all ten can be improved by strength training alone.

And strength training reduces fat and increases flexibility. In fact, Olympic weight lifters are second only to gymnasts when it comes to flexibility.

It also reverses age-associated change in the gene expression profile of skeletal muscles in aged humans—halfway back toward the young adult profile. Inactivity changes gene expression signatures from young to old. In other words, if done properly, weight training can make you young. Laziness will prematurely age you.

And finally, many published papers show resistance training is better than aerobic training for insulin resistance. As soon as you exercise a muscle, you increase its insulin sensitivity. Simple exercise increases the blood flow to that muscle. And one of the factors that determines insulin sensitivity is how blood can get there. It has been shown conclusively that resistance training increases insulin sensitivity.

How to Weight Train

Your best benefits do not come from doing a tremendous number of exercises. They come from the intensity of the sets you are doing. In other words, work to your peak performance. Quality, not quantity, of your exercises is what will give you the most out of your workouts. Work up to muscle failure if possible. Your last repetition is your most productive one.

In fact, you can DOUBLE your results this way. In other words, your last rep, if performed to complete muscle failure, is worth as much as the total of all the preceding reps in your set. So if your routine includes twenty sets, and if each rep lasts five seconds, you can double the effectiveness of your training session by adding a little more than a minute and a half to it.

Don't work the same body part to failure more than every two or three days. Muscles need rest to grow. So don't overdo it! You have 168 hours in your week. Devoting just three of those hours vastly improves the other 165.

Gradually work up to a good fitness level. Do your routine two to three times a week, stretch for flexibility at the end, and include a variety of exercises—or cross training. Cross training is a good idea for cardio exercise as well. You might integrate yoga or Pilates into your exercise program. They are great for energy, stamina and flexibility, and they help you avoid injuries. Or you might want to try the Tibetan Rites of Rejuvenation. These are 2500-year-old physical movements that some people say make you grow younger. You can see a demonstration by Ellen Wood of the correct way to perform them at www.howtogrowyounger.com/p/tror.html.

Follow these general guidelines for basic strength training:

- Do strength exercises for all your major muscle groups at least twice a week, but not for the same muscle group any two days in a row.

- Gradually increasing the amount of weight you use is the most important part of strength training.

- Start with a low amount of weight (or no weight), and increase it gradually.

- When you are ready to progress, first increase the number of times you do the exercise (repetitions or "reps"), then increase the weight at a later session.

- Do 8 to 15 reps (a "set"). Rest for a minute and do another set or two.

- Take 2 to 3 seconds to lift and 3 seconds to lower weights. Never jerk weights into position.

- If you can't do more than 8 reps, the weight is too heavy for non-advanced training. If you can do more than 15 reps, it's too light.

- When bending forward, always keep back and shoulders straight to ensure that you bend from the hips, not the waist.

Build Muscle, Not Size

Contrary to popular belief, strength training actually makes you smaller, not bigger. How's that? Because a pound of muscle is five times denser than a pound of fat, and therefore is five times smaller. This means a 150-pound woman with only 25 pounds of fat will easily fit into clothes that a 135-pound woman with 50 pounds of fat cannot. Since one pound of muscle takes as much space as five pounds of fat, resistance training can let you enjoy optimal health and make you look fantastic without losing weight—or even by gaining weight.

Would you be willing to swap thirty minutes a day to lose ten pounds of sloppy body fat for three pounds of lean, strong calorie-burning muscle? Then move more, and eat less.

If you're serious about becoming super fit in minimum time, if you want to maximize your training results, or if you are a competitive athlete, I strongly recommend you get a copy of *Ready, Set, GO! Synergy Fitness* by Phil Campbell.

I recently met Phil at Greta Blackburn's FitCamp in Malibu, Calif. Also on staff were two of the top personal trainers in the country. In fact, one of the world's biggest fitness equipment companies hired them to represent the company. They were secure with their abilities, and it was well-deserved confidence. Then they met Phil. They said it was a humbling experience and that they knew about twenty-five percent of what Phil knew.

If you're serious about fitness, get his book. Better yet, get to know him. His book taught me tons. His personal instruction taught me the world about training.

Cardio Training

Aerobic training's benefits are endless: improved breathing, more energy, improved heart health and cardiac output, lower blood pressure, decreased serum cholesterol, reduced stress, better sleep, improved mood and mental functioning, improved digestion and bowel function and more.

Increasing the health of your cardiovascular system comes primarily from aerobic exercise, and this has extremely beneficial effects on overall lifespan. If you recall from the above information, heart disease is the number one killer in the United States. Help avoid it with aerobic, or cardio, training.

A May 3, 2012 report from the Copenhagen City Heart study shows exciting longevity results from aerobic exercise. Between one and two-and-a-half hours of jogging per week at a 'slow or average' pace increases the life expectancy of men by 6.2 years and women by 5.6 years.

Your aerobic exercise should include activities such as running/jogging, bicycling, elliptical machines, stair-steppers, treadmills, brisk walking or swimming. It must significantly raise your heart rate for at least twenty minutes to get the maximal effect.

Note that extremely long periods of aerobic activity do not result in greatly enhanced cardiovascular health. In fact, even though you work up a good sweat and fatigue yourself, you may actually be depleting muscle and not fat. Interval training, like the *Sprint 8* that Phil Campbell teaches, is your key to maximum cardio health, muscle tone, speed, endurance and overall health.

We're not saying you should quit long-distance running if you enjoy it. It's just not necessary for excellent health and may be counterproductive. Any intense sustained exercise for over forty-five minutes could be detrimental, even if you want maximum growth. After about forty-five minutes of strenuous exercise, your body tends to cannibalize itself by using muscle tissue as an energy source. Also, long duration exercise causes your body to store fat rather than to burn fat.

Doing your aerobic exercise first thing in the morning on an empty stomach is a very effective way to burn fat. Your body is already depleted of its energy stores from the night before, so it must reach into its reserves (fat) to fuel aerobic activity. So if you are looking to lose a few pounds, work out first thing in the morning.

If you happen to be a die-hard weight trainer and don't enjoy any of the above activities, you can still get some benefit of aerobic training by lowering the rest time between each of your sets to sixty seconds or less. This will keep your heart rate high enough to get some of the same effects as aerobic exercise.

Resistance training with heavy weight and long rest periods in between sets will only give you strength and bone density benefits and not the cardiovascular benefits. In fact, there is some evidence that weight training without aerobic activity can actually increase your chances of a heart attack or a stroke. So if you prefer weight training, make sure you get some aerobic activity too.

Okay, so what types of cardio and weight exercise should you do to get these benefits, and when should you do them?

Ideally, you should exercise six to seven days a week for 20 to 45 minutes a session. If you train hard, take one or two days a week off for maximum benefits. A good mix of strength training and aerobic activity will provide the best combination of all the aforementioned health enhancements. You can exercise any time of the day you want, before eating, two hours or more after a meal and two hours or more before bedtime. Strenuous exercise will interfere with your sleep if you do it late at night.

Let's Get Started

Always begin your exercise session with at least five minutes of a warm-up exercise, which will bring your heart rate up to 50% of your maximum (see target heart rate in the next illustration). At the end of your workout, make sure you cool down by walking or continuing to perform your activity at a reduced rate for five to ten minutes. Tapering down speeds recovery, helps rid your muscles of waste and may be good for your heart.

Build up your endurance gradually, starting out with as little as five minutes of endurance activities at a time, if you need to. Starting out at a lower level of effort and working your way up gradually is especially important if you have been inactive for a long time. It may take months to go from a very long-standing sedentary lifestyle to doing some of the activities suggested in this section.

Your plan is to work your way up, eventually to a moderate-to-vigorous level that increases your breathing and heart rate. It should feel somewhat hard to you (level 13 on the Borg scale).

When you are ready to progress, build up the amount of time you spend doing endurance activities first; then build up the difficulty of your activities later. Example: First, gradually increase your time to thirty minutes over several days to weeks (or even months, depending on your condition) by walking longer distances, then start walking up steeper hills or walking faster.

The more exertion, the greater the benefits. Be sure to warm up and cool down with a light activity, such as easy walking. And your activities shouldn't make you breathe so hard you can't talk unless you are doing interval training. They shouldn't cause dizziness or chest pain.

Finally, stretch for five to ten minutes at the end of your workout when your muscles, ligaments and tendons are warm and lubricated. There are many reasons to be flexible. If you can't move well, all daily activities, fitness endeavors, athletic performance, strength training and general health can be compromised. Stretching, especially yoga, improves every other aspect of fitness and preserves your youth as much as anything.

Here's the conventional stretching technique: Breathe deeply, hold your stretch for twenty seconds minimum, and increase your stretch slightly on your exhale. Never stretch too hard. Only go to the point where you feel a mild pull. And do not bounce.

However, an increasingly popular technique is called active isolated stretching (AIS). It's supposed to be a breakthrough that helps you bolster your flexibility, improve flexibility faster and retain the gains you've made. In AIS, you hold a stretch for 1.5 to 2 seconds and do 6 to 8 repetitions instead of 10 to 30 seconds as you would in traditional stretching.

The perfect environment to stretch a muscle is when it's *relaxed*. AIS stretching avoids maximum effort, because overloading the stretch can cause microtears to a target muscle. The research concluded when a stretch is held for longer than two seconds, a protective mechanism called "myotatic stretch reflex" is triggered. This reflex happens in your body under many normal circumstances. However in elite performance, injury rehabilitation or the desire to instill lasting changes in the body, this reflex is undesirable.

By using repetitions, great amounts of lymph are moved through your body. This improves wound and injury healing as well as detoxification. Additionally, AIS is touted to result in an enhanced immune system and a reduction of aches and pains among other benefits.

Learn more about AIS at www.stretchingUSA.com.

One training aspect most people overlook is balance. Spend a few minutes a day improving it. One way to start is to hold onto a table or chair with one hand, and stand on one foot, then on the other. Then use one finger, then no hands. If you are steady on your feet, progress to no hands, and finally, to doing it with your eyes closed. You also might progress to doing one-legged squats if you are strong and supple.

Ask someone to watch you the first few times, in case you lose your balance.

Another way to improve your balance is through "anytime, anywhere" balance exercises. For example, balance on one foot, then the other, while standing during the day.

Intervals – Another Longevity Path

Rather than a long, steady low to medium intensity effort, consider interval training for twenty minutes or more. Interval training can burn up to nine times as much fat than sustained medium intensity exercise. Studies also show it promotes much greater cardiac fitness.

Interval training maximizes fat loss in minimum time, while reshaping your body with lean muscle. It burns up to 50% more calories, not just while you train, but for hours afterwards. For every pound of muscle you gain, you can burn 35–50 calories more per day with zero added effort. So if you add just one pound of muscle, you will burn up to 18,000 extra calories every year. That means you burn more calories—while you eat, sleep and relax. Adding four pounds of muscle burns as much calories as running two miles every day. How much fat does a pound of body fat burn per year? Only 700. Muscle also helps prevent diabetes, while making you look great twenty-four hours a day.

First warm-up for at least five minutes. Then do one to two minute sprints at 80–90% of your capacity. Then go through a recovery of one to two minutes at 40–50% of your capacity, and continue this cycle for twenty minutes. Do this routine three to six days per week. If you prefer longer drawn-out aerobic exercises, by all means, do those. The important thing is, get moving.

High intensity exercise though, is the gold standard for fitness… and longevity. It was recently endorsed by the European Society of Cardiology. A study conducted among cyclists in Copenhagen, Denmark showed it is the relative intensity, and not the duration of cycling, which is most important in relation to all-cause mortality. It's even more pronounced for coronary heart disease mortality. The study concluded that men with fast intensity cycling survived 5.3 years longer, and men with average intensity 2.9 years longer than men with slow cycling intensity. For women, the figures were 3.9 and 2.2 years longer, respectively.

This study suggests a greater part of the daily physical activity in leisure time should be vigorous, based on the individuals own perception of intensity.

In nature, arteries don't wear out, harden, clog or explode. It's inactivity that makes cardiovascular disease our #1 killer. Then throw in modern diets—and you create a perfect storm.

You now know the risk of developing cardiovascular disease, and type 2 diabetes is greatly reduced through regular physical activity. However, I'll bet you know people who feel they simply don't have time to follow the kind of training guidelines I suggest.

Enter Professor James Timmons and his research team at Heriot-Watt University Edinburgh, Scotland. They studied brief periods of high-intensity interval training (HIIT). Using sixteen sedentary male volunteers, they found doing a few intense exercises, each lasting only about 30 seconds, dramatically improves your metabolism in just two weeks.

The low volume, high intensity training utilized in their study substantially improved both insulin action and glucose clearance in otherwise sedentary young males. The volunteers exercised on stationary bikes, and the concept applies to most forms of exercise.

This is not as good as longer duration sessions, but it's *much* better than nothing. In fact, by doing just *three minutes* of High

Intensity Training (HIT) a week for four weeks, you could see significant changes in important health indices.

In fact, HIT may be the most effective all-natural approach to slow down the aging process by reducing telomere shortening. This is reinforced by other studies too. A nearly 5,000 person study from the Norwegian University of Science and Technology's K.G. Jebsen Center of Exercise in Medicine suggests that the greater the intensity of exercise, the higher your peak oxygen uptake will be and the longer you'll live. Those years won't just be tacked on either. You'll have less health problems and more vibrancy.

So tell your friends to get off their butts, if only for a few minutes a day. Research shows that relatively short bursts of intense exercise—even if done only a total of a few minutes each *week*—can deliver many of the health and fitness benefits you get from doing hours of conventional exercise.

While it's theoretically possible to reap valuable results with as little as three minutes once a week, it's more beneficial doing them two or three times a week for a total of four minutes of intense exertion per session, especially if you are not doing strength training. Doing it more frequently than three times a week can be counterproductive, as your body needs to recover between sessions.

Focus on making sure you're really pushing yourself as hard as you can during your two or three weekly sessions, rather than increasing the frequency. Intensity is the key for reaping all the benefits interval training can offer.

Lack of time is the number one reason people give for not exercising regularly. And lack of results, once they do start exercising, isn't far behind. Interval training every other day is a great solution for both of these common complaints.

In wrapping up, build up to all exercises and activities gradually, especially if you have been inactive for a long time. And if you have to stop exercising for more than a few weeks, start at half the effort when you resume, then build back up to where you were.

Measuring Your Activity

To gauge if you are getting the correct level of activity, there are two common scales currently in use. Target heart rate (THR) is the rate at 50–85% of your maximum ability. This range is where the maximum aerobic advantage is gained from the exercise. The chart below lists the desired target rates for different age groups for well-conditioned individuals who can work at 70–85% of their THR. A simple way to calculate your target heart rate is to subtract your age from 220, and multiply by the desired percentage.

The other method of judging the effectiveness of your workout is a subjective scale, known as the Borg Scale. Using this method you would determine the amount of work you are doing by the effort you feel from performing the exercise. For aerobic exercise, you should be in the moderate difficulty range or in the high difficulty range for your sprints if you do interval training. For strength training you should feel the exercise is in the high difficulty range. In order to grow stronger from exercise, your intensity has to be greater than your body is used to.

Target Heart Rates (70–85%)   Borg Scale

Target Heart Rates (70–85%)

Age	Desired Range for Heart Rate During Endurance Exercise (beats per minute)
40	126–153
50	119–145
60	112–136
70	105–128
80	98–119
90	91–111
100	84–102

Borg Scale

Effort		
Least effort		
6		
7	very, very light	
8		
9	very light	
10		
11	fairly light	ENDURANCE
12		TRAINING
13	somewhat hard	ZONE
14		
15	hard	STRENGTH
16		TRAINING
17	very hard	ZONE
18		
19	very, very hard	
20		
Maximum		

(Source: *Exercise: A Guide by the National Institute on Aging*)

Physical fitness doesn't have to be overly difficult. All you really need are basic strength and aerobic exercises to be in great shape. You don't need any fancy equipment—a good set of dumbbells can do wonders, but good equipment can make it easier and more fun. There are many excellent books on physical fitness if you need some suggestions on setting up a routine.

Find and do exercises that you enjoy. And never stop learning about fitness. The more you know about the positive benefits exercise gives you, the more naturally you will gravitate towards physical activity. The more you do, the better you will look, feel and function. Your energy level will shoot through the roof. Exercise will stop being something you know you ought to do and quickly become something you want to do.

This applies to diet and all seven steps in this book. Once you internalize this information and start looking for more, a healthy lifestyle will become a part of who you are. You will naturally gravitate toward health and away from obesity, faded looks and disease. When you exercise, everything works better. If you're not biologically 15–20 years younger than your chronological age, you are not all you can and should be. And you are cutting into your odds of capturing extreme health and open-ended longevity.

You can slow your aging down more than you think. Maximum Life Foundation has determined that diet and exercise alone could increase the average lifespan to over 90 years. Simply taking care of your life and your body might add over fifteen years to your lifespan if you start early enough in life. But it's never too late to start. Starting later still adds quality years.

So diet and exercise are the two most important things for you to master if your goal is optimal health, longevity and appearance. For maximum overall results, eat high-quality food within forty-five minutes of training.

How many people do you know whose plan is to get fat, out-of-shape and unhealthy and to shorten their lives? None, right? Yet how many run out and buy the biggest clearest television they can find? Then they buy the softest, plushest sofa or recliner they will fit into. Now they're on their way to accomplishing the exact opposite of what you know will keep them healthy. Why? Because rather than doing something active, they have figured out a comfortable way to spend their time. Also, people who watch television eat more food. And one more thing, watching TV downgrades their brain's cognitive function. But that's good, right? After all, if they turn themselves and their children into zombies, they'll be fat, happy and just won't care—at least not until their first heart attack.

If you know such a person, especially one who is important to you, wouldn't you want to share some of this information with him or her? The best expression of love could be to help another reach optimal health. So share what you have learned in this book with others. In fact, the best way to learn is to teach. By teaching health and wellbeing, you will gradually internalize this life-saving information until it becomes a part of who you are. Then you're on auto-pilot to a very long, happy and adventurous life.

Much of your fitness success stems from your attitude toward exercise. I have a separate chapter devoted to attitude, but for now here are some mindset tips to help you meet your fitness goals:

➢ Think about exercise.

➢ See yourself as healthy and fit.

➢ Think of exercise as fun.

➢ Associate (link) the negative effects of your bad habits to those habits.

➢ Celebrate small gains and victories.

Don't Forget Your Brain

Exercising your muscles also improves your brain function by making your neurons more robust while improving blood flow, oxygen and nutrients to your brain. But consciously exercising your brain is just as important as your body. Your brain atrophies through disuse, just like your muscles. Continue learning new things; play chess or other challenging games; do crossword puzzles; read and participate in problem solving. If you're right-handed, practice doing things with your left hand, and vice versa. Your rewards will be more vitality, greater alertness, enhanced thinking power, better retention, clarity of mind and insurance against dementia.

Here are five simple ways to maximize your brain power:

1. Fuel your body with good nutrition including targeted brain nutrition.

2. Exercise your body regularly.

3. Exercise your brain regularly.

4. Balance your hormones.

5. Reduce and manage stress in your life.

Now read on to see what else you can do to pave your road to open-ended youthfulness.

CHAPTER 7. STEP 3— NUTRITIONAL SUPPLEMENTS

Just twenty years ago, vitamin popping was still held by the mainstream medical community as a worthless fad. But studies now show we are woefully vitamin deficient. For example, two USDA surveys of 5,188 people and 16,103 people discovered that *not one* got 100% of the recommended daily allowances (RDA) for vitamins, minerals and nutrients. And RDAs are far below what many researchers determine to be optimal levels.

Today, you would be hard-pressed to find a physician who would disagree with the tremendous potential health benefits supplements can provide. That's because we finally have tens of thousands of published studies supporting the use of supplements. We also have ways to measure just what, if any, positive effects many supplements have on you. In fact, we now know you can fix defects in your DNA with vitamins and minerals.

According to the *Proceedings of the National Academy of Sciences* (PNAS), there are many genetic differences that make people's enzymes less efficient than normal, and that simple supplementation with vitamins can often restore some of these deficient enzymes to full working order.

There are over 600 human enzymes that use vitamins or minerals as substances that need to be present in order for a specific reaction to take place, and this study reports what they found by studying just one of them. This means even if the odds of you having a defect in only one gene is low, with 600 genes, you are likely to have some mutations that limit one or more of your enzymes. This report comes from the University of California, Berkeley.

Thanks to emerging technologies, we will soon be able to tell precisely what supplements and what dosages are optimal for you. For now, we need to take a more general approach.

According to Dr. Bruce Ames of the University of California at Berkeley, over fifty genetic diseases have already been identified that can be corrected by aggressive nutritional supplementation. Diet alone and recommended daily allowances (RDAs) will never do it for *optimal* health. In fact, optimal health is not possible without supplements for most of us. Thousands of studies support supplementation.

Dr. Michael Rose believes the best future strategy for radically extending human lifespans several-fold may be nutritional supplementation. In *The Future of Aging*, he states: "Evolutionary nutrigenomic agents can emulate the process of natural selection using nutritional supplements in lieu of genetic variation."

There has been a recent explosion in alternative medicine and herbal remedies. Many of these products and services have tremendous potential benefits, but many others are worthless. We will try to make some sense of this burgeoning industry and cover the most common vitamins, herbs, drugs and other supplements available to the consumer.

What Supplements Should You Take?

Science is far from perfect. Until we learn more, we'll have to understand what we already have to the best of our abilities. Although we know quite a bit about various supplements, there's much more that we don't know.

So do not follow anyone's advice blindly when it comes to your health. When determining what supplements you should take and how much to take, look for the most reliable studies on each supplement. There are five general classifications of medical studies. Here they are in order of the most reliable to the least reliable:

1. Long-term group studies where participants were randomly selected

2. Case controlled studies where one group has risk factors and the other group doesn't

3. Case series studies where there is no control group and where members of the group being studied share a specific disease

4. Animal studies

5. *in vitro* studies (studies performed in a dish or test tube

6. If the studies are independent of anyone having a vested interest in the outcome, they tend to be far more reliable than those being sponsored by an interested party. So pay attention to who paid for the studies. Do they have anything to gain from either outcome?

Published studies showed that supplementing with antioxidants can cut the risk of heart disease by 26–46%, as well as cutting risks from certain forms of cancer.

A cheap regimen of vitamins in use for decades is seen by scientists as a way to delay the start of Alzheimer's disease and dementia, a goal that prescription drugs have failed to achieve.

Supplementation can also help you avoid stroke, diabetes, arthritis, macular degeneration and much more. The bare basics include a daily high potency multi-vitamin tablet and essential fatty acids. Ninety-seven randomized trials involving over 275,000 subjects showed omega-3 fatty acids, like fish oil, reduced cardiac mortality risk by 32% and overall mortality by 23%.

The October, 2011 issue of *Life Extension Magazine* reports published studies show you can reduce your risk of dying prematurely from *all* causes by as much as 85% by maintaining optimal levels of omega-3 fats. If you aren't supplementing with at least 2 grams a day of a high-quality omega-3 product, you may be unnecessarily courting an early death.

The article goes on to say, studies show that daily doses of 1 gram or more of EPA and DHA significantly reduce scores on standard depression rating scales, especially in older adults. Omega-3s also have an anti-obesity effect. They improve insulin sensitivity and glucose tolerance, reduce blood pressure, lower triglycerides, can raise your HDL levels, protect your skin cells from cancer-causing effects of the sun, and can dramatically reduce the chances of breast cancer and even chronic kidney disease.

You may consider krill oil as an alternative to fish oil, because it contains potent antioxidants, and fish oil doesn't.

This could be a drawback for fish oil, because as you increase your intake of omega-3 fats by consuming fish oil, you actually increase your need for even more antioxidant protection.

That's because fish oil is pretty perishable, and that causes oxidation, which leads to the formation of the unhealthy free radicals we discussed earlier. Therefore, antioxidants are required to ensure that the fish oil doesn't oxidize and become rancid inside your body. So, you should take additional antioxidants when using fish oil. If your fish oil is encapsulated though, that should solve any potential rancidity issues. For the time-being, I prefer high-quality fish oil, at least until more independent studies support krill. You might consider taking both.

Know Your Omega Balance Score

A new and extremely important clinical test will set you on your way to optimal health. Unlike other blood tests that may be useful in one disease or area of your body, the Ideal Omega-3 Test gives information about every cell and every organ. The correct balance of Omega-3 and Omega-6 fatty acids is vital for optimal health. It is not possible to reach your true health potential if this balance is not right.

Many clinical studies have shown that correcting this Omega imbalance can act as an effective treatment for many of the chronic inflammatory conditions. Go to www.idealomegatest.com for information on this home test.

If you don't learn anything else today, go out and buy some high quality fish or krill oil capsules. Take 2,000 mg of fish oil twice a day with antioxidants. If you take krill oil, you won't need as much dosage.

Under your doctor's supervision, a daily baby aspirin (81 mg) or whole aspirin can reduce your risk of heart attack and stroke. According to The Nurses' Health Study at Women's Hospital in Boston, risk can be reduced by up to 50%. John Radcliffe Hospital in Oxford, England's study concluded whole aspirins or less can lower your risks of dying from many types of cancer, including:

- 40% lower risk of colon cancer

- 10% lower risk of prostate cancer

- 30% lower risk of lung cancer

- 60% lower risk of esophageal cancer

So if you're at risk and can tolerate aspirin, one of the most convenient and inexpensive ways to avoid serious disease is to take this 3¢-a-day supplement with your biggest meal.

Other basic supplements include coenzyme Q_{10}, carnosine, alpha lipoic acid, vitamin D3, a high-quality absorbable resveratrol, and folic acid. Folic acid may be more effective if you get it from whole foods, especially fresh, dark green vegetables. And most importantly, take glutathione—but only the "protected" form. Your best insurance against errors when your DNA gets copied is glutathione, which nutritionally supports normal cell replication. That happens 300 billion times every day! A protected glutathione product may soon be available. For current information, send an email to info@MaxLife.org.

You can and should feed your brain as well with many of the supplements above plus ginkgo biloba; A-L carnitine; PS (phospatidylserine); PC (phospatidylcholine); DMAE and EPA/DHA.

Some of these supplements, along with folic acid, some of the B vitamins and others enhance methylation.

Methylation is a chemical reaction, taking place millions of times a day, in every cell in your body. Your body depends on this biochemical exchange for some of its most critical functions, such as: detoxifying carcinogens and other poisons, repairing damaged DNA, forming new cells and manufacturing anti-aging hormones. (Hormones are the chemical messengers that control virtually every biological process in your body.) If your body doesn't methylate properly, you will travel the path headed for accelerated aging, heart disease, Alzheimer's, cancer, diabetes and other conditions.

Fortunately, it's easy to improve your methylation with supplementation. In fact, taking methylation-promoting nutrients is one of the primary preventable causes of aging and disease.

Also, if you or someone you know has arthritis, lymphoma, herpes, HIV, low energy, Parkinson's or frequent infections including colds and flu, these people may have a common link—nutritional deficiency. Researchers found that in almost any diseased condition, patients are glutathione deficient.

The supplements for which we have found the most supporting benefits and the most clinical data by far, are six key antioxidants. These six substances are vitamin C, vitamin E, coenzyme Q_{10} (CoQ_{10}), glutathione, lipoic acid and carnosine. Dr. Lester Packer of the University of California at Berkeley, one of the world's most renowned experts on antioxidants, has found the first five to act as an antioxidant network in your body.

One problem with antioxidants is once they detoxify a free radical (discussed in Chapter Three), they themselves become a free radical. In fact, vitamin C, a powerful antioxidant, can actually become a pro-oxidant (a free radical) and cause damage if it is not supported by other antioxidants. This is where the antioxidant network shines.

The combination of vitamins C, E, glutathione, CoQ_{10} and lipoic acid form a supporting network, according to Dr. Packer's studies. This allows each of the members of the network to recycle each other and prevent any formation of more free radicals. By detoxifying each other, they keep your ability to eliminate free radicals robust and healthy.

Reactive oxygen species (free radicals) play a direct role in heart disease, cancer, type 2 diabetes, strokes, Alzheimer's, Parkinson's, cataracts and arthritis. The advantages of having a great antioxidant system are many:

> Antioxidants, especially vitamin E and CoQ_{10}, have been shown to be effective in preventing heart disease.

> Antioxidants, both oral and topical, can prevent skin damage and rejuvenate older looking skin.

> Antioxidants enhance the effectiveness of your immune system.

> Antioxidants reduce all types of inflammation, and arthritis in particular.

> Antioxidants will slow brain aging and prevent memory loss and mental problems later in life.

> Antioxidants have been shown to improve concentration and focus.

When Should You Start and How Much Should You Take?

The age at which to consider supplementing is around 25. That's when the long term effects of nutritional scarcity start being felt. But supplementation really becomes essential by 40.

The daily requirements for each of these antioxidants as established by the USDA are far too low, according to the accounts of a large number of scientists and physicians. There is still a heated debate as to what the correct dosages should be, and they will vary from person to person. At present, the following guidelines are based on the general recommendations of Dr. Lester Packer.

Vitamin C, according to Dr. Packer, should be taken in doses of 250 mg, twice daily. According to the results from his work, any more is not going to do any harm if you have a well-supported antioxidant network. Above this amount though, much of it is just excreted in the urine without being used. Some people advocate taking mega-doses of vitamin C based on the reasoning that animals that produce it naturally make two to three times as much under conditions of stress and that it has extraordinary health benefits. Notable researchers such as Dr. Linus Pauling, Dr. Thomas Levy and Dr. Robert C. Cathcart, as well as a 1995 Hoffman La-Roche study, found that up to 10 grams per day is safely utilized by the body.

The USDA recommended daily allowance (RDA) for vitamin E is woefully low. Vitamin E is one of the frontline defense systems against free radicals. Dr. Packer and many other sources recommend a total of 500 mg (733 I.U.) of vitamin E per day, and higher dosages for people with cancer or heart disease. Dr. Packer and others recommend mixed natural tocopherols and tocotrienols, members of the vitamin E family.

Premature aging is one primary side effect of having too little CoQ_{10}. This essential vitamin recycles other antioxidants such as vitamins C and E. CoQ_{10} deficiency also accelerates DNA damage. And because CoQ_{10} is beneficial to heart health and muscle function, this depletion leads to fatigue, muscle weakness, soreness and eventually heart failure.

CoQ_{10} is naturally found in nearly every cell, tissue and organ in your body. It is found in especially high concentrations at the source of most of your free radical production, the mitochondria, your cells' "power plants." It improves your cells' ability to transport electrons in and out of the mitochondria. CoQ_{10} is especially attracted to high energy organs such as your heart and brain. It directly recycles vitamin E and is one of the primary molecules in the energy production system of cells. As we age, the production of CoQ_{10} declines, and this may be a factor in heart disease as well as diminished cellular energy.

The antioxidant action of the reduced form of CoQ_{10} (ubiquinol) is now considered to be one of its most important functions in cellular systems. Ubiquinol is a potent antioxidant capable of regenerating other antioxidants and provides important protection against oxidative damage to fats, proteins and DNA. Recent studies also reveal its function in gene expression involved in human cell signaling, metabolism and transport.

Many recent studies point out that plasma ubiquinol declines in response to neurodegenerative disease, cancer, fatigue and especially Type 2 diabetes, in addition to cardiovascular disease.

The ubiquinol acts as an important first-line defense against the oxidative insult associated with these diseases.

If you take ubiquinone instead of ubiquinol, make sure it is the water soluble form. It may be just as effective at a much lower cost.

If you are in the older and/or are in a disease/stress category, you may want to start at 200 to 300 mg per day. Studies show the CoQ_{10} plasma levels plateau at about two to three weeks at this dose. A good maintenance dose after that is in the 50 to 100 mg per day range. Make sure you take ubiquinol, the reduced form or water soluble ubiquinone. Other forms are easily oxidized and are therefore inefficient.

The February, 2011 issue of *Life Extension* Magazine reports on the newest companion product to CoQ_{10}. It is pyrroloquinoline quinone, or PQQ. Early in 2010, researchers found it not only protects your mitochondria from oxidative damage, but it stimulates growth of *fresh* mitochondria!

The implications of this are huge! PQQ protects your brain, heart and muscles against degenerative disease. It is also shown to optimize health and function of the entire central nervous system and may be a potent intervention in Alzheimer's Disease and Parkinson's Disease. In addition, it has the potential to *reverse cellular aging* by forming new mitochondria in aging cells.

PQQ is a master antioxidant and is now classified as an essential nutrient. Daily recommended dose is 20 mg. Coupled with 300 mg of CoQ_{10}, it may even *reverse* aging-related cognitive decline in humans.

A low level of glutathione is one of the key indicators for premature death. Unfortunately, the body breaks down glutathione in the digestive tract. So supplementing with an unprotected version of glutathione won't do you much good. However, as I previously indicated, there is now a protected version of glutathione. Another way to keep your glutathione levels up is to avoid nitrates found in processed lunchmeats, smoking and alcohol. Supplementing with N-acetyl cysteine (NAC) may increase your levels as well.

More on Antioxidants

In addition to the five key antioxidants found in your body, there are other compounds that can boost your antioxidant activity. One group of these molecules that has gotten a lot of attention as of late is the flavonoids. These antioxidants are found in tea, berries, red wine and many fruits.

From recent studies, flavonoids seem to act as free radical scavengers, mainly recycling vitamin C. This appears to have a very positive overall effect on the antioxidant system. Two of the most powerful flavonoid antioxidant extracts are those from pycnogenol (pine bark) and ginkgo biloba.

Most of the mental and sexual enhancement effects felt by people taking ginkgo is probably from the ability of flavonoids to improve circulation and allow better chemical signaling to occur. In addition to these benefits, the antioxidant effects mentioned above are enhanced. Dr. Packer's recommendation for ginkgo biloba is 30 mg daily and for pycnogenol, 20 mg daily.

Another group of antioxidants available from plant, algae, and fungi are the carotenoids. The best source of carotenoids is your diet. Brightly colored fruits and vegetables all contain high levels of these compounds (see Chapter Five, Nutrition). These molecules are also available in capsule form. Conventional wisdom says if you are eating a diet with five to seven servings of vegetables and one to three servings of fruit a day, this is probably not necessary (one serving equals one-half cup).

However, conventional wisdom may be wrong. The fruits and vegetables we eat today may only contain a fraction of the nutrients they contained fifty years ago. Many soils have been depleted of minerals, and in their attempt to sell food that looks and tastes good and keeps from spoiling too early, the industry has adulterated much of our produce. We recommend you eat as much locally grown or organically grown food as possible for those reasons, and because organic foods generally contain far fewer toxins. And oh yes, I believe organic food tastes better too.

How do you know whether or not the food you buy that is labeled "organic" is truly organic? The term is becoming so popular that many food companies use the term loosely. Look for food that is labeled "100% organic." If it's labeled "Certified Organic", that means it must be at least 95% organic. If you don't see either of these designations, be wary. Buying from small local farms or farmers' markets may be your best bet then, especially if you get to know the farmers.

Conventional wisdom also leads to "normal" health. For "optimal" health, we suggest supplements.

Wide Range of Benefits

Additionally, recent studies show vitamin D does far more than promote healthy teeth and bones. Its role in supporting immunity, modulating inflammation, and preventing cancer make the consequences of vitamin D deficiency potentially devastating. A growing number of scientists who study vitamin D levels in human populations now recommend annual blood tests to check vitamin D status.

University of California recently conducted an extensive review of scientific papers published worldwide between 1966 and 2004. Their analysis suggested that taking 1,000 international units (IU) of vitamin D3 daily lowers an individual's risk of developing colorectal cancer by 50%. And a new European study suggests vitamin D supplements could prolong your life. "The intake of usual doses of vitamin D seems to decrease mortality from any cause of death," said lead researcher Dr. Philippe Autier, from the International Agency for Research on Cancer in Lyon, France.

In fact, people with the lowest blood levels of vitamin D were about two times more likely to die from *any cause* during an eight-year study period than those with the highest levels.

If vitamin D3 levels among populations worldwide were increased, 600,000 cases of breast and colorectal cancers could be prevented each year, according to researchers from the Moores Cancer Center at the University of California, San Diego (UCSD). This includes nearly 150,000 cases of cancer that could be prevented in the United States alone.

Another study shows getting about 2,000 IU to 4,000 IU a day of vitamin D can help you to reduce your cancer risk by up to 50%! And according to Dr. William Grant, internationally recognized research scientist and vitamin D expert, about 30% of cancer deaths, which amounts to 2 million worldwide and 200,000 in the United States, could be prevented each year with higher levels of vitamin D.

Furthermore, in the September, 2011 issue of the *European Journal of Clinical Nutrition,* W. B. Grant of the Sunlight, Nutrition and Health Research Center in San Francisco concludes that doubling one's serum level of vitamin D from 54 to 110 nanomoles per liter might increase life expectancy by an average of two years.

Here's a mechanism which may explain vitamin D3's life extending capabilities:

Daily supplementation of only 2,000 IU of vitamin D3 significantly increased telomerase activity in overweight African Americans. The study suggests vitamin D3 may improve telomere maintenance and prevent cell senescence and counteract obesity-induced acceleration of cellular aging. This was published in the International Journal of Obesity advance online publication on October 11, 2011.

Just as scientists are discovering critical new roles for vitamin D, they are also finding that shockingly few people have blood levels of vitamin D adequate to support their daily needs. Most people only get 250–300 IU a day from their diet, so another source, ideally the sun, is essential. Because vitamin D3 is obtained primarily from exposure to sunlight, this puts people living outside the tropics at particular risk for vitamin D deficiency, especially from late fall to early spring. The elderly may be more prone to vitamin D deficiency as well, since vitamin D does not get manufactured very efficiently by older skin. University of California at San Diego, researchers have found an association between lower sun exposure and higher Type I diabetes rates in children, which they attribute to vitamin D levels.

Further compounding the problem, many public health officials are concerned that their warnings about avoiding the sun because of skin cancer risk may in fact be causing people to limit their sun exposure to an unhealthy extent.

Many scientists and physicians consider sunlight as food for the body, brain and eyes. Researchers have shown that when our skin is exposed to the sun's rays, a compound is released in our blood vessels that helps lower blood pressure. The findings suggest that exposure to sunlight improves health overall, because the benefits of reducing blood pressure far outweigh the risk of developing skin cancer.

Production of this pressure-reducing compound, called nitric oxide, is separate from the body's manufacture of vitamin D, which rises after exposure to sunshine. Scientists say it's the sun's UV rays that lead to health benefits, which also explains why dietary vitamin D supplements alone will not completely compensate for lack of sunlight.

Taking vitamin D by itself orally is unnatural, and it is possible to overdose over prolonged periods of time. So be sure to take the natural D3 version. Consider measuring your vitamin D3 level with your regular blood tests if you take high-doses. Make sure you get the most accurate test, 25(OH)D. You want to measure your results against optimal levels, not normal levels.

Be cautious with overexposure to the sun as well, but it's hard to overdose on vitamin D3 from the sun. For prolonged exposure during peak hours, use a good sunscreen from most health food stores, at www.lef.org/maxlife or at www.life-enhancement.com. Avoid most commercial sunscreens. They may be toxic. You can find sunlight protocols at www.mercola.com.

Vitamin K

According to Dr. Cees Vermeer, one of the world's top researchers in the field of vitamin K, nearly everyone is deficient in vitamin K—just like most are deficient in D.

Most people get enough K from their diets to maintain adequate blood clotting, but NOT enough to offer protection against some health problems.

Vitamin K comes in two forms, and it is important to understand the differences between them before devising your nutritional plan of attack.

1. **Vitamin K1:** Found in green vegetables, K1 goes directly to your liver and helps you maintain a healthy blood clotting system. It is also K1 that keeps your own blood vessels from calcifying, and helps your bones retain calcium and develop the right crystalline structure.

2. **Vitamin K2:** Bacteria produce this type of vitamin K. It is present in high quantities in your gut, but unfortunately is not absorbed from there and passes out in your stool. K2 goes straight to vessel walls, bones, and tissues other than your liver.

You can obtain all the K2 you'll need by eating 10-15 grams of natto daily, which is half an ounce. The next best thing is a vitamin K2 supplement. Remember to take your K supplement with fat, since it is fat-soluble and won't be absorbed without it.

Although the exact dosing is yet to be determined, Dr. Vermeer recommends between 45 mcg and 185 mcg daily for adults. Use caution with higher doses if you take anticoagulants. Even though the risk of increased clotting tendencies may be small, it is real.

In 2004, the *Rotterdam Study*, which was the first study demonstrating the beneficial effect of vitamin K2, showed that people who consume 45 mcg of K2 daily live seven years longer than people getting 12 mcg per day.

Vitamin K and vitamin D work together to increase MGP, or Matrix GLA Protein, which is the protein responsible for protecting your blood vessels from calcification. And the results of human clinical studies suggest that concurrent use of vitamin K2 and vitamin D may substantially reduce bone loss. We may be seeing just the tip of the iceberg when it comes to vitamin K and its many valuable functions in your health.

Astaxanthin

Scientists long ago discovered that carotenoids held powerful antioxidant properties that are crucial for your health. These are the compounds in your foods that give you that vibrant cornucopia of color—from green grasses to red beets, to the spectacular yellows and oranges of bell peppers—as well as all of the beautiful flowers in your garden.

Recently, one particular carotenoid jumped to the front of the line in terms of its status as a "supernutrient," becoming the focus of a large and growing number of peer-reviewed scientific studies. This carotenoid is called natural astaxanthin and is now thought to be the most powerful antioxidant found in nature.

There are only two main sources of astaxanthin—the microalgae that produce it, and the sea creatures that consume the algae (such as salmon, shellfish, and krill).

What Makes it so Special?

There are many properties that make this carotenoid unique. Here are the main differences:

Astaxanthin is by far the most powerful carotenoid antioxidant when it comes to free radical scavenging. It is 65 times more powerful than vitamin C, 54 times more powerful than beta-carotene, and 14 times more powerful than vitamin E.

Astaxanthin crosses the blood-brain barrier *and* the blood-retinal barrier (beta carotene and lycopene do not), which brings antioxidant and anti-inflammatory protection to your eyes, brain and central nervous system and reduces your risk for cataracts, macular degeneration, blindness, dementia and Alzheimer's disease.

➢ Astaxanthin is soluble in lipids, so it incorporates into cell membranes.

➢ It's a potent UVB absorber and reduces DNA damage.

➢ It's a powerful natural anti-inflammatory.

➢ It protects your cell membranes and DNA from oxidative damage.

➢ It improves visual acuity and depth perception.

> ➤ It improves sun tolerance and reduces your tendency to sunburn.

> ➤ Astaxanthin improves strength and endurance.

Use only *natural astaxanthin*, not the synthetic version.

Breakthrough Longevity Supplement

A new anti-aging product called StemCode™ has recently been introduced. I have been testing it for over a year, and I'm impressed.

I tried it before it hit the market, because I'm familiar with the 27 years of genomic research behind it. That research showed aging is linked to altered expression in more than a hundred genes. The lab discovered this by studying long-lived animal assays to screen for wide-spectrum herbal extracts that extend lifespan. They succeeded in greatly extending animal lifespan using a novel class of nutrigenomic supplements that fine-tune genes involved in both aging and age-related disease.

After I had been taking the product for two months, I found out it increases both average and maximum life span in lab animals, even when started at middle age. As far as I know, it is the only supplement proven to double the lifespan of an animal model. I have not seen any other supplement come close.

Effects vary among individuals. But the general expectation is, for most health measurements that are in the normal range for your age, StemCode can promote readings you had when you were 20 years younger. I believe this supplement alone may have the potential to add at least five quality years to your life.

I have been fortunate. Most of my biomarkers are in healthy ranges, and I have been doing a lot for many years to get them and keep them there. Even so, since taking this product, my already good blood glucose level dropped by 11% since my previous reading, and my HDL level increased slightly, even while my total cholesterol dropped by 5%. My LDL level dropped by over 11% as well. When total cholesterol drops, you would expect both HDL and LDL to drop accordingly. So my results are positive.

The main effects that have been observed in their clinical tests are: lower blood pressure, somewhat lower LDL and higher HDL and reduced fasting blood glucose. Expect to see lower blood pressure and blood glucose within two weeks of taking StemCode if they are elevated. The cholesterol changes will take longer. Check after two months.

The scientists also believe telomere loss will be reduced with the supplement due to lower stress levels and reducing both oxidative damage and inflammation.

Besides the changes in lab tests, some have seen other anecdotal advantages such as more endurance during vigorous workouts, reduced anxiety levels, elevated mood, cleared sinuses and lost belly fat. Longer term, some have observed improvement in their gum health, less eye stigmatism, and smoother, more elastic skin.

You can see what else StemCode can do by visiting www.MaxLife Solution.com.

You may or may not feel any different within a month when taking any anti-aging supplement—even one that works. Statins and baby aspirin are two examples of drugs with apparent anti-aging characteristics that typically lack any feel-good aspects. Yet, both drugs have lowered all-cause mortality in large scale clinical trials. If you are already in excellent health, you may not observe any real difference with treatment unless you monitor the silent biometrics of lipids, blood pressure and glucose. These biometrics are the best known indicators of future lifespan and healthspan.

Round out Your Program

There are two more compounds worth mentioning in this discussion: selenium and melatonin. Selenium is an element that has a synergistic effect on the antioxidant network. The way it works is not completely clear yet, but it is well known that selenium deficiencies are responsible for higher levels of heart disease and cancer. In fact, people who live in areas in which the soil is selenium deficient are much more likely to die of heart disease. Dr. Packer recommends taking 200 mcg (micrograms) per day.

Melatonin is technically a hormone, so it might actually belong in Chapter Eight (Anti-Aging Medicine). But one of its most powerful uses is as a general antioxidant. This molecule has the ability to cross the blood-brain barrier, the membrane that prevents most molecules from entering the brain itself. So this might be one of the brain's key defenses against oxidation.

In addition to these effects, melatonin has a role in regulating the sleep cycles of some animals, and may have similar effects in humans. Melatonin production declines with age in humans, and so it has been suggested that increased dosages may be necessary as you age. The most commonly recommended dosage is 3 mg or less at night before bed, but this is an unusually benign substance. Dosages up to 1,000 mg have been taken by humans in experiments. The only noticeable side effect was it is hard to wake up in the morning. Of course this is extreme, and we don't recommend extreme dosages of anything.

We feel uncomfortable suggesting any particular dosages for various supplements. We're all physiologically unique. One size does not fit all. For optimal health, and before starting any aggressive supplement protocol, see a qualified anti-aging physician. It could be the best investment you ever made or will make.

Here are some general dose ranges though. Don't be intimidated by the number of supplements in this chart. Nearly half can be found in a good multivitamin/mineral supplement, and other products can combine several others.

Supplement	Recommended Daily Dosage
Vitamin A	4000 IU
Vitamin B1	100–500 mg
Vitamin B2	25–100 mg
Vitamin B3 (Niacin)	100–500 mg
Vitamin B5	100–2000 mg
Vitamin B6	50–100 mg
Vitamin B12	100–1000 mcg

Vitamin C	500–2000 mg
Vitamin E (mixed tocopherols – Alpha/Gamma)	200–400 IU
Vitamin D3	5000–8000 IU
Vitamin K (menaquinone-7)	100 mcg
Acetyl-L-Carnitine	500–2000 mg
Alpha lipoic acid	100–300 mg
Anthocyanins	100–500 mg
Aspirin	81 mg
Astaxanthin	3-12 mg
Betacarotene	2500–5000 IU
Carnosine	1000 mg
Calcium (from dicalcium malate or bis-glycinate)	1000–1200 mg
Coenzyme Q_{10} (ubiquinol)	50–300 mg
Copper	1–2 mg
Chromium	400–800 mcg
Curcumin (Super Bio-Available)	400–1200 mg
DHEA	15–50 mg
Digestive enzymes	
Fish oil	1400 mg EPA/1000 mg DHA
Folic acid	400–800 mg
Flavonoids	50–100 mg
Flax Seed	1–2 tablespoons
Garlic (Kyolic)	600–1200 mg
Gingko Biloba	60–100 mg

Ginseng Root	250–500 mg
Glutathione	50–200 mg
Grapeseed extract	50–200 mg
Green tea extract (99%)	500–1000 mg
L-arginine	2–9 grams
L-cysteine	500 mg
Magnesium	400–800 mg
Manganese	3–10 mg
Melatonin	0.5–10 mg
Phosphatidylcholine	1200–2000 mg
Phosphatidylserine	100 mg
Potassium	500 mg
PQQ	20 mg
Probiotics	20–500 mg
Resveratrol	250 mg
SAM-e	200–1600 mg
Selenium	100–400 mcg
Zinc	30–75 mg

Although my personal dosages are generally higher, I suggest you have an anti-aging specialist monitor your blood panels, as I do, if you get aggressive with supplementation. I often wonder if I overdo it. The answer is, I don't know. Once we can affordably map personal genomes and learn what to do with all the data, we'll have a much better idea. Until then, much of what we take advantage of is educated guesswork.

I buy almost all of my supplements from Life Extension. I have been a member of Life Extension Foundation (LEF) for twenty-five years. Here is their list of the twelve most important supplements you can take if you want to simplify your longevity protocol.

1. Life Extension Mix (in my opinion, the world's most complete and most potent multi-vitamin/mineral formula)

2. Super Omega EPA/DHA with Sesame Lignans and Olive Fruit Extract

3. Vitamin D3

4. Super Ubiquinol CoQ$_{10}$

5. Mitochondrial Energy Optimizer

6. Restoring Youthful Hormone Balance (see an anti-aging physician or speak to one of LEF's consultants)

7. Cognitex (a brain booster and protectant)

8. Bone Restore

9. Ultra Natural Prostate with 5-Loxin® and Standardized Lignans (for men)

10. S-adenosylmethionine (SAMe)

11. Low Dose Aspirin

12. Super Booster Softgels with Advanced K2 Complex

I follow all of these recommendations and have for years. If you decide to join LEF, or to buy products from them, please say Maximum Life Foundation sent you. If you do, part of all the money you invest in their supplements will be donated to MaxLife, a non-profit foundation, to invest in life extension research and development.

If you wish to find further information about any of the supplements we have discussed here as well as others, please look to the following sources.

➢ Life Extension Foundation, www.lef.org/maxlife, a not-for-profit organization that donates proceeds of the sale of supplements to anti-aging research. This group is a highly reliable producer of reasonably priced and high-potency pharmaceutical grade supplements and a terrific source of current health and research information.

➤ Ray Kurzweil and Terry Grossman's Health Products, www. rayandterry.com. Also, review their Longevity Program, described in their book, *Fantastic Voyage: Live Long Enough to Live Forever*. They illustrate how heart disease, cancer, stroke, respiratory disease, kidney disease, liver disease, and diabetes do not appear out of the blue. They are the end result of processes that are decades in the making.

➤ MaxLife Solution, www.MaxLifeSolution.com. This is a website that benefits Maximum Life Foundation and is owned by Age Reversal, Inc. So far, MaxLife Solution has identified several research-based products that have proven life extending capabilities.

MaxLife'sTop 8 Supplements

If you want an even more streamlined list for basic yet potent longevity purposes, here is what we recommend you take on a regular basis:

1. Bioavailable glutathione
2. High quality fish oil
3. D3
4. High potency multi vitamin/mineral
5. Telomerase activators—see www.MaxLife.org/telomeres for breaking news.
6. PQQ
7. InflaGene if chronically inflamed, overweight or over age 50
8. StemCode

Maximum Life Foundation's advisors estimate the top three cost about $55 per month and could potentially slash healthcare costs in half. That means a savings in the U.S. of up to $1.2 trillion a year; year after year, after year. The cost to supplement the 250 million adults would be about $165 billion annually. That comes out to a net annual savings of over $1 trillion—plus the benefits of increased productivity and less suffering. Good return on investment, don't you think?

Is anyone awake in Washington?

But What About the Anti-Supplement News Articles I See?

I could write a whole chapter on this issue alone. Instead, let me lay some groundwork for you and also give you an example.

The FDA and international government agencies have been trying to regulate supplements for many years. And they have made inroads in spite of the fact that people take over 60 billion doses of legitimate vitamin and mineral supplements per year in the USA without a single fatality. Not one.

In striking contrast, drugs are known to cause well over 125,000 deaths per year when taken correctly as prescribed. And the U.S. National Poison Data System's annual report tracked data from 57 U.S. poison centers. The report showed vitamin and mineral supplements caused zero deaths in 2010, while pharmaceuticals caused more than 1,100 of the total 1,366 reported fatalities.

If vitamin and mineral supplements are allegedly so "dangerous," as the FDA and news media so often claim, then where are the bodies? Why are dietary supplements under so much attack?

There are legitimate concerns over unscrupulous profiteers who adulterate weight loss and body building supplements with banned substances. But instead of enforcing existing laws, regulators continue trying to impose broad reaching restrictions on the entire industry.

It's no secret that the industry is big, growing and profitable. And the drug industry took notice. In some ways, dietary supplements are a threat to their business. In another way, they see a profit opportunity. They are already getting into the supplement business. Don't you think they'd love to have a monopoly like they do with drugs?

You decide.

Now here's a recent example of a news article attacking nutritional supplements. Two studies, a rehashed review, and an editorial published in the December 17, 2013 issue of the Annals of

Internal Medicine have attempted to discredit the value of multi-vitamin supplements.

Both of the studies were plagued by grievous methodological flaws.

In one of the studies, subjects were given low-quality, low-potency multivitamin supplements. Treatment adherence rates and drop-out rates were horrendous. Nevertheless, mainstream sources are using these slanted studies to undermine dietary supplements.

The first study examined the cognitive effects of low-potency multivitamin supplementation in aging male participants. In the other study, subjects with a history of heart attack were given a multivitamin supplement or placebo and monitored for about 4.5 years for cardiovascular events. Despite succumbing to obvious *design flaws*, this study actually revealed evidence that multivitamins reduced cardiovascular risk. However, the investigators constructed the study so as to ignore anything short of miraculous cardiovascular risk reduction, so the conclusion drawn questions multivitamin benefits.

Subjects in the first study were considered to have adhered to their multivitamin regimen appropriately if they took it just two-thirds of the time. In other words, even subjects who skipped their multivitamin **4 months** out of the year were deemed "adherent" to the intervention.

In addition, the method by which adherence was assessed in this study is inherently weak. The multivitamin utilized in this study contained woefully inadequate nutrient concentrations. Even the researchers state a limitation of their study is "[the] doses of vitamins may be too low…"

Despite the low potency vitamins used in this trial, benefits were seen in the multivitamin group.

In the cardiovascular event study, a staggering **46%** of subjects discontinued the multivitamin regimen during the study. Despite concluding that multivitamins don't protect against cardiovascular risk, the investigators did find an **11%** reduction in their primary endpoint (composite of time to death from any cause, heart attack, stroke, coronary revascularization or hospitalization for angina) among those taking multivitamins.

But in this study, the authors designed the trial to eliminate 1 in 4 cardiovascular event outcomes.

By setting the bar for efficacy so high, this study was set up to conclude that multivitamins would provide no benefit from the outset.

You can find a full report at www.lef.org/featured-articles/ Flawed-Research-Used-to-Attack-Multivitamin-Supplements.htm.

Cancer Caution

Much of what you do for longevity may be counterproductive if you have cancer. For example, some supplements may feed your cancer cells right along with your healthy cells. All the other steps in this book are recommended for cancer patients, with your doctor's supervision. But if you have cancer, I strongly suggest you visit Dr. J. William LaValley's Website before you supplement. See www.integrativeoncologywellnessplan.md. Dr. LaVally is one of the few medical doctors in the world with a deep understanding of what effect, good or bad, certain supplements could have on cancer patients.

His information may help you and your physicians increase the effectiveness of the treatment they give you. It may also help protect your healthy cells and reduce the harsh side effects of chemotherapy and radiation without interfering with the desired benefits of those therapies. Dr. LaValley has a spectacular track record of adding lots of quality life to terminally ill cancer patients.

The Most Effective Cancer Cure on the Planet

According to the Associated Press, smoking is responsible for about 30% of all cancer-related deaths. Obesity ranks second, at 14% and 20% for men and women, respectively. As you browse the seven steps in this book, you can see how many controllable factors contribute to the vast majority of cancers.

So doesn't it make sense that the best way to keep from becoming a victim is prevention? Then why do so many people ignore this simple strategy? Laziness, denial, inertia? The simple fact is you can avoid most cancers. And if you do get cancer, your most effective path to cure is catching it in its early stages.

Adopting the seven step protocol in this book will improve your odds dramatically. You have more than a 35% chance of becoming a cancer victim if you follow the crowd and don't take preventative measures.

Most victims don't know they have it until it's too late for effective treatment. Once you show symptoms, the cancer may have been growing inside you for years. Symptoms are often a death sentence with painful agonizing treatment offering you the most hope. Sometimes the treatment is worse than the disease. Cancer is a nasty mess that you want to avoid or detect early at all costs.

So my second best advice is to have your cancer detected early if you do get stricken. Stage I cancer survival rates are excellent, about 90%. Stages III and IV are a dismal 10%. So see your physician for early warning signs. Most cancers are hard to detect until you see symptoms though, and then it may be too late. That's why prevention is critically important. Currently, the Canary Foundation and others are hard at work developing sophisticated early detection tests such as blood biomarkers samples and ultrasound imaging.

Breast Cancer

Mammograms pose significant and cumulative radiation risks, especially for premenopausal women. Even worse, false positive diagnoses as high as 89 percent are common, leading many women to be unnecessarily and harmfully treated by mastectomy, more radiation or chemotherapy.

There are instances where mammography may be warranted. But other more effective, less expensive, and completely harmless diagnostic tools are available.

Imagine being able to look inside yourself and get as much as *ten* years warning that something is *about* to develop, *before* any tumors have formed. Now you have time to *prevent* the cancer from forming in the first place by taking the appropriate lifestyle changes outlined in *Smart, Strong and Sexy at 100?*

That technology is Thermographic Breast Screening, a safer, more effective alternative. It simply measures the radiation of infrared heat from your body without using mechanical pressure or radiation. It can even detect the potential for cancer.

Compare that to a mammogram that can't detect a tumor until after it has been growing for years.

Number three advice is to get the best treatment you can find and afford whether you have early or late-stage cancer.

From time-to-time, we discover validated nutritional supplement breakthroughs. If you would like to be among the first to be notified when they are released, please go to www.MaxLifeSolution. com and www.MaxLife.org/sssbook.

The next chapter opens your eyes to the way your doctor should be treating you now and how medicine will be practiced in the future.

Chapter 8. Step 4—Anti-Aging Medicine

M ost doctors are simply mechanics. They do their best to fix you when something goes wrong, if it's not too late. Anti-aging medicine may fix you, too. But more importantly, it helps ensure something doesn't go wrong with you in the first place. A good anti-aging specialist could keep you from needing a mechanic. (Did you ever notice most people take better care of their cars than they do of their own bodies? It's sad but true. It's also insane.)

I recommend having an anti-aging specialist as your primary physician. If he or she is not an internist, find a good internist too, in case something goes wrong and you ever need treatment. Modern medicine usually equates to treatment over prevention. If you work with a good anti-aging physician, though, you'll need only a fraction of the modern medicine our society has come to rely on.

Imagine, first, people make themselves sick. Then they compound their woes by subjecting themselves to medical procedures. According to an article in the prestigious Journal of the American Medical Association (JAMA), doctors are the *third* leading cause of death in the United States! Doctors cause 225,000 deaths per year. Here is JAMA's breakdown:

- 12,000 – unnecessary surgery

- 7,000 – medication errors in hospitals

- 20,000 – other errors in hospitals

- 80,000 – infections in hospitals

- 106,000 – non-error, negative effects of drugs

You can avoid 90% of this risk by applying what you learn here, including seeing a preventative medicine specialist.

A good anti-aging doctor will start with an extensive blood panel to evaluate your present condition and to establish a baseline for you. He or she will recommend colonoscopies every 5–10 years after the age of fifty or sooner (this alone could reduce your colon cancer death chance by 90%), will schedule other important tests and will monitor your health and progress. If you're over fifty and never had a colonoscopy, you're playing with your life.

Contact Life Extension Foundation if you would like an affordable source of blood tests. See www.lef.org/maxlife.

The Ten Most Important Blood Tests

1. Chemistry Panel and Complete Blood Count
The Chemistry Panel and Complete Blood Count (CBC) is the best place to begin your disease-prevention program. This low-cost panel will give you and your physician a quick snapshot of your overall health. This test provides a broad range of diagnostic information to assess your vascular, liver, kidney and blood cell status.

2. Fibrinogen
An important contributor to blood clotting, fibrinogen levels increase in response to tissue inflammation. Increased fibrinogen levels can help predict the risk of heart disease and stroke and other inflammatory disorders such as rheumatoid arthritis.

3. Hemoglobin A1C
This test measures a person's blood sugar control over the last two to three months and is an independent predictor of heart disease risk in persons with or without diabetes.

4. DHEA
Dehydroepiandrosterone (DHEA) is frequently referred to as an "anti-aging" hormone.

5. Prostate-Specific Antigen (PSA) (Men Only)
Elevated levels may suggest an enlarged prostate, prostate inflammation, or prostate cancer.

6. Homocysteine
High homocysteine levels have been associated with increased risk of heart attack, bone fracture and poor cognitive function.

7. C-Reactive Protein
C-reactive protein (CRP) is a sensitive marker of systemic inflammation that has emerged as a powerful predictor of coronary heart disease and other diseases of the cardiovascular system.

8. Thyroid Stimulating Hormone (TSH)
When blood levels fall below normal, this indicates hyperthyroidism (increased thyroid activity, also called thyrotoxicosis). When values are above normal, this suggests hypothyroidism (low thyroid activity). Undiagnosed mild disease can progress to clinical disease states. This is a dangerous scenario, since people with hypothyroidism and elevated serum cholesterol and LDL have an increased risk of atherosclerosis. Have your Free T3 and Free T4 measured as well.

9. Testosterone (Free)
Testosterone is produced in the testes in men, in the ovaries in women, and in the adrenal glands of both men and women. Men and women alike can be dramatically affected by the decline in testosterone levels that occur with aging. Test also for Total Testosterone.

10. Estradiol
In women, blood estradiol levels help to evaluate menopausal status and sexual maturity. Increased levels in women may indicate

an increased risk for breast or endometrial cancer. Estradiol plays a role in supporting healthy bone density in men and women. Low levels are associated with an increased risk of osteoporosis and bone fractures in women and men as well. Elevated levels of estradiol in men may accompany gynecomastia (breast enlargement), diminished sex drive and difficulty with urination.

Other Tests

*   Annual urinalysis to check for diabetes, kidney disease or infection warning signals

*   Body fat percentage

*   Fat-free mass

*   Hydration

*   Basal metabolic rate

*   Body mass index

*   VO$_2$ max to tell you how much oxygen you are extracting from a given volume of air. It measures your lung health, the amount of hemoglobin in your blood and your heart's pumping ability.

You can get these additional tests at physical therapists' offices, sports medicine clinics or at human performance labs.

Early detection will save you suffering and money... and could save your life.

Hormone Replacement Therapy

Most anti-aging physicians use hormones to treat aging. After reviewing available data, we currently feel proper hormone replacement therapy (HRT) can be extremely beneficial to those over the age of fifty, who are experiencing declines in their hormone levels.

Here's our rationale for this conclusion. We mentioned in the introduction that, as we age, we have certain control systems that begin to break down. One set of these key systems are those parts of the brain (the endocrine system) that control the level of hormones circulating in your body.

For reasons that aren't completely clear yet, these systems start to go out of balance in middle age, resulting in a steady decline or sometimes an abrupt shutoff in production of particular hormones. Since medical science has yet to come up with a way of turning these systems back on in humans, the next best thing is to try to manually regulate our hormonal levels.

One of the major concerns with HRT, and especially estrogen, was that it might increase a person's chance of having cancer. In the case of breast cancer, this idea has been greatly exaggerated. There is little or no data in human beings that shows "natural" estrogen increases the chances of cancer. (There are studies that show evidence of serious health problems caused by "synthetic" forms of estrogen.)

But natural estrogen has so many benefits for aging women, it should be worth exploring. Consider this: Approximately half of all women die from heart disease, and less than 10% die from breast cancer. In fact, pre-menopausal women rarely get heart attacks. Natural estrogen has been shown to be very protective against almost all forms of heart disease and provides terrific protection against osteoporosis. So if you are a woman, you have a 50% chance of dying of heart disease, or a 10% chance of dying of breast cancer.

For men, there also happens to be very little data to support the idea that testosterone will cause prostate cancer. In fact in some studies, it has been shown to possibly protect against it. The problem is that if you do have prostate cancer there are two kinds—one that is made worse by testosterone and the type that isn't affected either way by it. So If you have a blood test and discover your testosterone levels are low, we suggest supplementing with testosterone under a qualified physician's guidance, but *only* after testing for prostate cancer (with a PSA test and a digital rectal exam). If your PSA is at all questionable, your physician might even suggest a transrectal ultrasound guided biopsy.

DHEA

The most commonly physician-supplemented hormones are estrogen and progesterone in women, testosterone in men, and growth hormone in both sexes. In addition to these hormones, the majority of people also experience a decline in the hormones melatonin and DHEA.

DHEA promotes tissue renewal and replacement. Low DHEA levels affect your cardiovascular and immune system as well as your metabolism. DHEA usually declines from prime levels by 80–85% by the time you reach seventy years of age.

DHEA is available as an over-the-counter supplement at any health food store. Have your physician recommend a sensible dosage for you. Dosages will vary from person to person.

Once again, the potential benefits of hormone replacement outweigh the negative consequences. These benefits include increased muscle tone, a more active sex drive, better skin and hair condition and better immune system function.

The important thing to keep in mind though is, when you incorporate HRT into your regimen, do so only under the guidance of an intelligent anti-aging physician. He or she should test your hormonal levels and monitor your health before and during supplementing hormones to make sure you aren't receiving too much. As with any biologic molecule, too much can be just as problematic as too little. The idea is to bring your system back into balance, not to overwhelm it.

A final word of advice about hormone replacement is that many people sell what they claim to be human growth hormone or human growth hormone releasing drugs. The majority are snake-oil salesmen. Be wary before purchasing any of these products. Many are completely unproven, and the companies that sell them usually can't be trusted. We are wary of growth hormone for anti-aging purposes no matter what the source.

See an Anti-Aging Physician Now

Many people look at old age as a decrepit, miserable period in their lives. The grumpy ones have for the most part given up hope.

For example, a colorful man lost his will to live. Here is an aging former soldier of fortune who once had a zest for life experienced by few. Now, he has lost interest in eating and seemingly everything else.

This bothers me for a couple of reasons. First, children may lose their dad. And on a larger scale, didn't I say most people go to the ends of the earth to hang on to life towards the end? Well, apparently not all. Why is this?

Several months ago, I had a relevant conversation with a close friend about how some people cling to life at the end no matter how much suffering and pain they endure, while others simply throw in the towel. We concluded it may have something to do with declining hormone levels. So I called my anti-aging physician to discuss this possibility. His response was that yes, declining hormone levels lead to depression, which usually translates to loss of appetite, and of course, a diminished will to live. He routinely reverses this phenomenon with closely monitored hormone replacement therapy.

Could declining hormone levels be evolution's way to nudge us into going quietly into the night? Could savvy doctors reverse deteriorating attitudes and improve and extend millions of lives with simple HRT?

The evidence strongly points in that direction.

The moral to this story is, don't wait until you see serious decline to visit an anti-aging specialist. In fact, see one before you experience any decline—period. After all, once you see signs of a condition or disease, it may be too late. Heart disease and cancer are two good examples. They eat away at you for years before you show symptoms. And one symptom from heart disease is often sudden death.

Your perfect cure is prevention.

There are many anti-aging clinics popping up around the country. We are seeing more and more physicians who specialize in anti-aging medicine. One of the primary treatments these physicians prescribe is hormone therapy. Most of these doctors are reputable, but some aren't. You might go to www.MaxLife.org and see the Medical Advisory Board. Some of the best qualified anti-aging physicians in the country are listed there with links to their excellent websites.

Another resource to find an anti-aging physician or health practitioner in your area is the American Academy of Anti-Aging Medicine. See their directory of specialists at www.worldhealth. net/pages/directory. Or call them at 866-693-3376. Or go to www. acam.org for a list of certified physicians in your area.

Be sure your physician makes every effort to track your progress through frequent lab tests and doesn't just prescribe hormones at random. Just because he or she displays a wall full of certificates, doesn't mean they are qualified to give you the best care. This is true for any medical specialist. To determine how well qualified your anti-aging physician is, ask him or her, the questions found at www.grg.org/resources/localmds.html.

An Easier Way to Get the Best Care

There's an old joke that is more tragic than funny. "What do you call the person who graduates last in his or her class at medical school?"

"Doctor"

I have had the good fortune to know some of the best anti-aging physicians in the country. I also met some of the worst. This specialty, just like every other, and every other profession for that matter, has its stars and its losers. But the big winners or losers are the consumers, and in this case, the patients. You.

Good doctors can change your life for the better... or for the worst. They can perform miracles and save your life, but they can also kill you. Doctors, unlike any other professionals, bury their mistakes.

So when it comes to something as precious as your health, how do you know whom to pick as your physician? As I mentioned, if you want a top anti-aging doc, you can go to www.MaxLife.org and pick one of our Medical Advisory Board members if you are lucky enough to live near one of them. If not, and this goes for most of you, I may have your answer. I have never met anyone who knows more about the human body, or how to diagnose and treat as wide a variety of ailments, as one individual.

About nine years ago, I met Professor Joe Carrington. Whenever I have a personal health issue, and especially when I want to maintain peak health, Joe is my go-to guy. I do have a primary physician, and Joe works with him when needed. Otherwise, I rely on Joe. He is a research scientist and pioneer in Holistic and Clinical Nutrition. He has focused his career in anti-aging medicine and diseases of aging with emphasis on neuro-degenerative conditions. Harvard University skipped him over two college degrees and admitted him directly into Harvard's Master's program. Professor Carrington practiced Clinical Nutrition for forty-three years, solving problems for many patients who could not be helped by their regular mainstream physicians. He jokes that he has no life, spending his time devouring every anti-aging book and article he could lay his hands on that was published over the past fifty years. Now here's how Joe can help you get better medical care, regardless of where you live.

He does not diagnose or prescribe. He would consult with you by phone, working hand-in-hand with your physician in getting you prescriptions for blood panels, other diagnostics and possibly medications which he would review with you and/or your physician. Here's his email address: carrington@post.harvard.edu.

Are Prescription Drugs Good for You or Bad For You?

Here's some breaking news about fish oil. The European Society of Cardiology reported a 2008 Italian study found omega-3 fatty acids to be superior to an Rx cholesterol-reducing drug. It showed fish-oil supplements work slightly better than the popular cholesterol-reducing drug Crestor in helping patients with chronic heart failure. This is just one of many examples of how natural treatments are just as, or more, effective than drugs, but without the side effects.

So let's talk a bit about conventional medicine—especially the chronic use of drugs to treat symptoms such as high blood pressure, high cholesterol, headaches, weight gain, etc. One example, weight loss drugs have the worst record of all drugs in terms of side effects and success rate. In 1977, a research project showed a modified diet consisting of eight to ten servings a day of fruit and vegetables lowered blood pressure as well as drug therapy.

Symptom treating may mask and actually increase the underlying causes. In almost all cases, if you treat a symptom you are going to make the disease worse. The symptom is there as your body's attempt to heal itself. Medication almost always causes an imbalance to your system. Most medicines are blunt instruments, and no one really knows what they'll do once they're inside of you. So the deadly paradox of chronic drug use can often deceive you into thinking you are doing your body favors, when in fact you may be masking the cause and sabotaging your biochemistry. You could be playing with deadly medicine—short-term gratification that costs you long-term health and satisfaction.

The predatory medical practice of borrowing from Peter to pay Paul can simply compound your problem. Do you know how big a vested interest the medical and drug industries have in keeping you sick and keeping you on medications? Why do you think they spend twice as much on advertising as they do on research? Sure, drugs can be life savers. Drugs and nutrients can both cure and prevent disease. But only pharmaceuticals have government sanction. And big pharma protects its turf.

Here's a useful report from www.Mercola.com that sheds more light on this topic:

> One of the best-kept statistical secrets in medicine is called "number needed to treat," or NNT.
>
> Most clinical trials look at how much better people do on a particular medicine. NNT answers the question: How many people have to take a particular drug to avoid one incidence of a medical issue (such as a heart attack, or recurrence of cancer)? For example, if a drug had an NNT of 50 for heart attacks, then 50 people have to take the drug in order to prevent one heart attack.
>
> That doesn't sound like a lot, so pharmaceutical companies tend to keep the number quiet and focus on broader statistics. But that could be changed if you ask for the NNT up front the next time you're handed a prescription.
>
> NNT was intended to help you make a decision about whether or not to take a drug. After all, having it put in simple terms

such as "Out of every 50 people who take this drug, perhaps one heart attack will be prevented, and the other 49 people will receive no benefit," puts things into perspective—a perspective that the drug companies do not want you to see.

One of the most blatant examples of how drug companies have hidden NNT for their own self-serving purposes lies with cholesterol drugs. These drugs, which can cause side effects like liver damage, muscle weakness, cognitive impairment and many others, are touted as miracle pills that can slash your risk of a heart attack by more than one-third.

Well, *Business Week* actually did a story on this very topic, and they found the real numbers right on Pfizer's own newspaper ad for the cholesterol-lowering drug Lipitor.

Upon first glance, the ad boasts that Lipitor reduces heart attacks by 36%. But there is an asterisk. And when you follow the asterisk, you find the following in much smaller type:

"That means in a large clinical study, 3% of patients taking a sugar pill or placebo had a heart attack compared to 2% of patients taking Lipitor."

What this means is that for every 100 people who took the drug over 3.3 years, three people on placebos and two people on Lipitor had heart attacks. That means that taking Lipitor resulted in *just one fewer heart attack* per 100 people.

The NNT, in this case, is 100. One hundred people have to take Lipitor for more than three years to prevent one heart attack. And the other 99 people, well, they've just dished out hundreds of dollars and increased their risk of a laundry list of side effects for nothing.

Not to mention that this study was funded by the industry, which means their results may already be skewed, and the actual benefit may be even *less* than what they found.

The NNT for some cholesterol-lowering drugs has been figured at 250 and up, even after taking them for five years!

Wow! Eye-opening, isn't it?

Do you know how America's health compares to other countries? Not too well. Yet we consume 50% of the world's prescription drugs. The other 95% of the world's population takes the rest.

That would be a good testimonial for drugs if we led the world in health and longevity. But we don't. We lag behind almost every other developed country. In fact, according to a Global Burden of Disease study, we are ranked a pathetic twenty-ninth in the world for male longevity and thirty-third for females. Don't buy into the story that you have to live on medications for lifestyle-related diseases. Statistics prove otherwise.

So keep thinking "cause" and not "symptoms." Take drugs when necessary. They can be life savers. But avoid chronic use unless you are well informed and well advised. The few hours you invest over time could reward you with revitalized health and extra years to appreciate it.

Unconventional Therapies for Cancer

We at Maximum Life Foundation predict that in just a decade or so, our current medical technologies of drugs and surgery will seem very barbaric. There are hundreds of different broad-based technologies and thousands of exciting breakthroughs being developed while you're reading this. Humans already have neural implants and the artificial pancreas; robotic hands can be connected to the brain; we have grown meat in a laboratory and cloned animals.

Another example, using strands of genetic material, Purdue University scientists have constructed tiny delivery vehicles that can carry anticancer therapeutic agents directly to infected cells, offering a potential wealth of new treatments for chronic diseases.

Or imagine a Trojan horse-like cancer drug that can burrow into a tumor, seal the exits and detonate a lethal dose of anti-cancer toxins, all while leaving healthy cells untouched. MIT researchers have designed a nanoparticle to do just that.

The way in which medical science currently treats many life-threatening diseases is similar to trying to rid your house of cockroaches with a hand grenade. For a long time, physicians have relied on these tried and true "brute force" techniques to battle cancer, heart disease, diabetes, etc.

Slowly but surely though, biomedical researchers are beginning to give doctors the tools to intelligently combat these diseases. It is no longer good enough just to fight the symptoms of a disease. Now we have the tools to understand how and why a disease works the way it does.

Therapy for cancer patients has actually changed very little in the past thirty years. The most commonly prescribed treatments are still to cut it out, burn it with radiation or kill it with chemicals. The problem with these ideas is that cancer cells are a part of the patient, so these therapies often cause tremendous collateral damage to the patient.

Newer techniques are being developed and applied that specifically target cancer cells where they live and breathe—in the very molecules that allow them to grow with such great speed.

There is an enzyme called cyclooxegenase II (COX-2), which many types of cancer cells produce in great quantities. Cancer cells use this enzyme to greatly speed up their metabolism, which in turn allows tumors to grow faster. Luckily COX-2 is also involved in rheumatoid arthritis, so drugs that have been developed for those patients may have great benefit for cancer patients. These drugs are called COX-2 inhibitors. To get these drugs, you will most likely have to get your physician to prescribe them for you. Some of the brand names of these products are Celebrex, Vioxx, Lodine XL and nimesulide, a European drug that is not yet approved by the FDA but is safer than any of those currently prescribed in the U.S. Both Celebrex and Vioxx have been linked to patient deaths. We prefer a natural COX-2 inhibitor, the supplement curcumin.

Another type of proteins that are typically over expressed in cancer cells are a group collectively known as the RAS oncogene family. These proteins are part of the normal signaling mechanism that cells use to control their reproduction. When there is too much of this type of signaling, cells divide too rapidly, growing out of control.

There is a group of cholesterol-lowering drugs that have been shown to stop the RAS proteins from signaling. This class of drugs is known as the "statins." One of these drugs is called lovastatin and has shown to be very effective is slowing the growth and spread of cancer cells.

A new type of drug still in clinical testing is also showing tremendous progress in fighting cancer growth. In order to grow, cancer cells need a blood supply just like any other cell type. Tumors have the ability to grow new blood vessels in order to feed themselves. This new class of drug stops the formation of new blood vessels, essentially starving the tumor. The two drugs currently undergoing testing are named angiostatin and endostatin.

And finally, how's this for an unconventional cancer therapy? Lifestyle!

Lifestyle actions are proven to activate telomerase and/or lengthen telomeres, including nutrition, exercise, and stress management techniques such as meditation, yoga, and deep breathing exercises. A landmark Dr. Dean Ornish/Dr. Elizabeth Blackburn 2008 pilot study following thirty cancer patients showed that targeted lifestyle actions led to a 29% increase in telomerase activity in 24 patients after only three months! Dr. Elizabeth Blackburn was awarded the Nobel Prize in Medicine in 2009 for the discovery of how chromosomes are protected by telomeres and the enzyme telomerase.

A newer Ornish study, published in the November, 2011 *The Lancet Oncology,* found lifestyle changes (similar to the recommendations in this book) significantly increase telomerase activity.

The long telomere proteins protect the ends of chromosomes in the body, but they shorten naturally and ultimately die unless the telomerase enzyme acts to repair them and increase their length. The association between the patients' extremely healthy habits and the increased amount of telomerase proved highly statistically significant.

Maintaining optimal telomere length is perhaps the hottest anti-aging topic in the world. Avoiding causes of telomere shortening should be one of your major longevity goals. Telomere length may be the most powerful biological clock that has yet to be identified. So prevent short telomeres as best you can.

The field of telomeres offers an enormously exciting and viable possibility for extreme life extension—the kind of anti-aging strategy that can actually allow you to regenerate and in effect "grow younger." there's solid evidence that simple lifestyle strategies and nutritional intervention can do this.

As published in *The American Journal of Clinical Nutrition* Volume: 89, Issue: 6, researchers found that women who use vitamin B12 supplements have longer telomeres than those who don't. Vitamin D3, zinc, iron, omega-3 fatty acids, and vitamins C and E also influence telomere length. This supports the findings of an earlier study from 2009, which provided the first epidemiologic evidence that the use of multivitamins by women is associated with longer telomeres.

Thousands of studies have been published on telomerase, and it is well-known to maintain genomic stability, prevent the inappropriate activation of DNA damage pathways, and regulate cellular aging.

Animal studies have shown that many types of health problems can be *reversed* by restoring telomerase functioning. They include:

- Decreased immune response against infections
- Type 2 diabetes
- Atherosclerotic lesions
- Neurodegenerative diseases
- Testicular, splenic, intestinal atrophy
- DNA damage

To optimize your telomere health, "telomere shortness" is the key, not "telomerase activation." Any and all interventions to forestall telomere shortening should be used, including: activating telomerase; reducing oxidative stress and lowering inflammation. For example, oxidative stress can reduce telomerase activity by 50%, and it accelerates the rate of telomere shortening, as does inflammation.

So look for "full spectrum telomere length," vs. just telomerase activation. For the latest breaking news on the best products that can help do this, periodically check www.MaxLife.org/telomeres.

By focusing on overall telomere length and preventing critical telomere shortness, you also incorporate the latest telomere science for preventing cancer, as backed by Dr. Blackburn.

A Brand New Tool

I often describe to people how you can widen your window of opportunity to take advantage of tomorrow's extreme life-extension technologies. These "bridges" could be the difference between your suffering and dying according to actuarial predictions... or enjoying an open-ended youthful lifespan. Some is out of your control, but you have a choice to dramatically improve your odds. Boarding the Longevity Express is such a choice.

The latest anti-aging medicine weapon in your arsenal is having your genomic profile read. Doing so could give you insights into what your particular genetic hazards are. Then you might be able to take steps today to reduce your risks. And get this: some experts in the field believe we could increase our healthy lifespans by at least ten years with this tool.

Now here's some really interesting news. The company providing this personal genotyping service for only $99 is 23andMe. www.23andme.com. The FDA however has recently determined that this type of information should be taken out of patients' hands and made the exclusive domain of the medical profession. Updates will be on the 23andme website.

That wraps up our chapter on medicine. Your longevity largely depends on staying informed. If you haven't done so already, subscribe to my newsletter, Longevity News Alert. I email it to you approximately once a week. You'll be able to keep up with breaking research news by investing a few minutes a week.

To subscribe, go to www.MaxLife.org. It's informative, it could be life saving, and it's free. So subscribe now.

Now that you know what your doctor should be doing for you, go to the next page to see what mistakes most people make and why those mistakes are killing them.

Chapter 9. Step 5—Lifestyle

Personal Decisions Are The Number One Cause of Death...

...Says Professor Ralph L. Keeney of the Fuqua School of Business at Duke University. He conducted a study where he analyzed the relationships between personal decisions and premature deaths in the U.S.

His analysis indicates that over one million of the 2.4 million deaths in 2000 can be attributed to personal decisions and could have been avoided if readily available alternative choices were made.

Dr. Thomas Perls says: "Many people assume that without those protective genes, we don't have a good shot at longevity," But the Adventist study shows that that's just not true."

Seventh Day Adventists are forbidden to smoke, drink, or eat meat. They are encouraged to exercise regularly and pray frequently. And almost all of them live into their 80s and 90s.

So, what this really means is that our health, and our death, is largely our own responsibility and of our own doing.

In short, lifestyle trumps genetics!

Do you need more convincing? Calculations show that about seventy percent of premature death is lifestyle-related. Generally speaking, any death prior to the late '80s should be considered premature, and we should be able to avoid at least 70% of the pain and suffering leading up to death from aging.

This does not even take into account emerging life extending technologies.

There's a lot of crossover between this chapter on lifestyle and several of the others. It's more corroboration than anything, yet there are specific items in this chapter that stand alone. Let's illustrate the corroboration with excerpts from a recently published article.

A study conducted by Dean Ornish, MD, of the Preventive Medicine Research Institute in Sausalito, California, along with researchers at the University of California, San Francisco, found that lifestyle improvements have a beneficial effect on gene expression in men with prostate cancer. The finding was reported in the June 17, 2008, issue of the *Proceedings of the National Academy of Sciences.*

> For a three-month period, participants were asked to limit dietary fat to 10% of daily calorie intake, adopt a whole-food, plant-based diet, engage in 30 minutes per day of walking for six days a week, and practice stress management in the form of stretching, breathing, meditation, imagery and relaxation for 60 minutes per day in addition to a one-hour per week group session. Diets were supplemented. Cardiovascular disease risk factors, including weight, body mass index, waist circumference, blood pressure, lipids, and C-reactive protein, were measured before and after the intervention.

> Gene expression in initial prostate biopsies was compared with prostate tissue samples obtained after three months of the lifestyle changes. Forty-eight genes, including those that have disease-preventive effects, were found to be up-regulated, and 453 genes, including oncogenes involved in breast and prostate cancer and other disease-promoting genes, were down-regulated following the intervention. Body mass index, blood pressure, lipids and waist circumference significantly improved. Benefits of the regimen were also observable in the participants' mental health-related quality of life and levels of cancer-associated mental distress.

Other studies have shown that just ten minutes of walking turns on a gene that reduces cancer growth rate, and that the nutrient resveratrol turns on a gene that slows or stops a dangerous inflammatory process. Inflammation ages your entire system.

This means lifestyle changes, the recommendations you get in this book, influence your genes in a positive way. Science's most sophisticated tools prove that a healthy diet, exercise, supplements and the way you manage stress all turn your important genes on or off in the right direction! It's been proven time and time again that if you don't reach the point of no return, you can take charge of your body and convert it from a state of degeneration to a state of regeneration. Your destiny is in your hands. This is NOT controversial stuff. It works! It keeps you alive! It makes you healthy!

Lifestyle and Your Heart

According to the American Heart Association, 1.3 million coronary angioplasty procedures were performed in 2006 at an average cost of $48,399 each, or more than $60 billion; and 448,000 coronary bypass operations were performed at a cost of $99,743 each, or more than $44 billion. Americans spent more than $100 billion in 2006 for these two procedures alone.

Despite these costs, a randomized controlled trial published in April 2007 in The New England Journal of Medicine found that angioplasties and stents do not prolong life or even prevent heart attacks in stable patients, or 95% of those who receive them.

Coronary bypass surgery prolongs life in less than 3% of patients. So, insurers and individuals pay billions for surgical procedures that are usually dangerous, invasive, expensive and largely ineffective. Yet they pay very little, if anything at all, for integrative medical approaches which have been proven to reverse and prevent most chronic diseases that account for at least 75% of healthcare costs.

The Interheart study, published in September 2004 in The Lancet, followed 30,000 men and women on six continents and found changing lifestyle could prevent at least 90% of all heart disease.

Let this sink in.

The disease that accounts for more premature deaths and costs Americans more than any other illness is almost completely preventable simply by changing diet and lifestyle. And the same lifestyle changes that can prevent or even reverse heart disease also help prevent or reverse many other chronic diseases as well.

Common Sense and Safety

Wouldn't it be tragic if you followed all of the advice in this book and then managed to electrocute yourself by sticking your finger in an electric socket to see if it were working? As we mentioned in the first section, accidents are the fifth highest cause of death in the U.S. Half of those deaths are automobile fatalities. If biomedical science succeeds as we at Maximum Life Foundation believe it will, twenty years from now, accidents will be the number one killer.

Advancing technology comes with a price. If you were able to go back in time and tell the leading developers of the automobile that their invention would be responsible for the deaths of millions of people, would they have continued? Here are some general notes on driving with safety:

➢ Never drive while incapacitated. Do not drive under the influence of any mind-altering substance and do not drive when overtired. Recent studies indicate a sleepy driver is just as dangerous as a drunken one.

➢ Be aware of the driving conditions, and drive accordingly.

➢ Maintain your car as if your life depended on it. It does. Brakes and tires should be inspected regularly.

➢ Always be aware of where vehicles are around you in all directions (i.e., check your mirrors and blind spots frequently).

➢ Drive defensively. The other drivers are usually not looking out for you, so look out for them.

Household accidents also rank high on the list of accidental causes of death. Survey your home for potential sources of accidents. Walk from room to room. Make immediate corrections if possible, and make a list of those things you can't do right away. Where are those sharp corners in your home? Those slippery floors? Dangerous items? Many people die each year from slips and falls in their own bathroom. Below are some other safety considerations.

➤ A fire extinguisher should be easily available in the kitchen.

➤ Every room should have a smoke detector.

➤ Keep all of your emergency numbers programmed in or next to a phone.

➤ Always read labels of household chemicals before using. Are they flammable? Poisonous?

➤ Be careful when mixing household chemicals. They can sometimes produce toxic fumes (ammonia and bleach, for example).

➤ Replace your toxic household cleaners, soaps, hygiene products, air fresheners, bug sprays, lawn pesticides and insecticides with non-toxic alternatives.

➤ Use any products that give off fumes in a well-ventilated area.

➤ Don't store household chemicals near an open flame or a heat source.

➤ Don't use or store toxic substances around food.

➤ Never take or administer medication in the dark.

➤ Never use medicine that is out of date, or that has crumbled or changed color.

> ➢ Always read the instructions for household appliances, especially for power tools.

> ➢ Be aware of unsafe electrical connections.

> ➢ Use ladders with great care.

> ➢ Lock and safely store firearms.

> ➢ At least one person in the household should be first aid and CPR certified.

> ➢ Finally, install a reliable home security system, if you don't already have one. And get a loud dog to discourage would-be intruders.

In general, simply be aware of your situation at all times. The most avoidable deaths are the ones caused by downright stupidity. That includes reacting to aggression or stupidity with your own aggression and stupidity, such as when someone cuts you off when you are driving. Why increase your odds of physical harm or even death over nothing? Save your aggression only for when your life is in danger and there is no other way out. You can be vigilant without being paranoid.

These suggestions will make your life safer.

Environmental Concerns

After the food in our diet, the next largest sources of damage to our bodies are the air we breathe, the water we drink and excessive exposure to radiation. In this section we will briefly outline ways to make sure you minimize your exposure to these sources of damage.

If you are a smoker, I'm sure you are sick and tired of hearing about how dangerous smoking is. Well we're going to tell you one more time. Smoking is *the* largest preventable underlying cause of death in the world. Did you know over 30% of all cancers are caused by tobacco? In fact, a September 14, 2011 Associated Press article said that according to the World Health Organization, 20% of *all* deaths in the world are linked to tobacco use.

Smoke from cigarettes has over two hundred individual carcinogens. So if you read this book but continue to smoke, forget everything else we have told you, because it won't do you much good unless you quit immediately.

Smoking breaks down your collagen and wrinkles your skin prematurely. Smoking not only makes people die young, but it also makes them look and feel old. Study after study proves smokers die over eight years sooner than non-smokers on average. In fact, 50% of smokers are eventually killed by their habit. Hmm, 50%. Heads you win. Tails you die.

Even if you win, you lose. If your genetic makeup keeps smoking from killing you, it doesn't keep smoking from destroying your lungs. Every regular smoker suffers lung damage.

And newer data from the U.S. Centers for Disease Control and Prevention shows that adult male smokers lost approximately 13.2 years of their lives and female smokers lost 14.5 years of their lives because of smoking. So is it eight years or 14 years? Either way, it's a serious killer.

Plus, chronic diseases caused by smoking tended to curtail the quality of life of smokers while they were still alive. According to the National Institute of Health and Medical Research in Villejuif, France, smoking in middle age is now even associated with memory deficit and decline in reasoning abilities. It's also a major factor behind asthma and allergies, and it aggravates stomach ulcers and heartburn. If that's not enough, smoking increases the risk of Alzheimer's, blindness, fractures and osteoporosis, blood clots in your legs, poor wound healing, increases impotence, and it makes you ugly.

But there's Good News for Many Smokers

According to an October 25, 2012 release by the *British Medical Journal,* a study showed that men born between 1920-45 who started smoking before age 20 lost nearly a decade of life expectancy. They had more than double the death rate of lifelong non-smokers, again suggesting that more than half of these smokers will eventually die from their habit.

Results on the few women studied who had smoked since before age 20 were similar. In addition to studying the risk of smoking, the researchers were able to examine the benefits of stopping. As elsewhere, those who stopped smoking before age 35 avoided almost all the excess risk among continuing smokers, and even those who stopped around age 40 avoided most of it.

I know it can be tough to quit, but people do it every single day. Over time, it becomes easier and easier to stay smoke-free, and you become better and better.

The best way to quit smoking is to go "cold turkey." Studies have shown that simply cutting back on how much you smoke does nothing to lower your cancer risk. So once you decide to quit, complete abstinence is required.

If you quit smoking and still eat an unhealthy diet, you may be tempted to replace the cigarettes with some other "reward." When that reward ends up being junk food, smokers gain an average 10 to 12 pounds after they quit. So stick to a healthy diet if you want to benefit from quitting smoking.

As bad as smoking is, that one French fry is almost as bad for you as one cigarette. So trading your pack a day for an extra fast food meal a day is a *bad* swap.

Some smokers get depressed after quitting, which makes it tough to make any major dietary changes and improvements to your health.

However, your new wholesome lifestyle is more likely to provide you with the incentive needed to quit. There's something about eating well and exercising that synergistically help to resolve the underlying anxiety that many people choose to resolve with smoking. And if they eat the right foods and exercise, it is very unusual for them to remain smokers.

Another common source of airborne damage to the human body is exhaust fumes from automobiles and their associated chemicals. If you exercise outdoors, stay away from busy streets. Because of increased respiration during exercise, you are even more likely to inhale noxious chemicals. Be aware that some of the additives found in gasoline (especially the one that causes that particular odor at the gas station) are known carcinogens.

The second largest cause of lung cancer in the U.S. is a radioactive gas that is found in many households throughout the country—radon. Radon is a colorless, odorless gas that can be deadly in high concentrations. It seeps up from the ground and sometimes becomes trapped in houses. You should make sure your house is tested yearly for radon, and possibly consider installing radon detectors and vents.

Another simple way to maintain air quality in your house is by installing air filtration units. People with allergies will certainly appreciate the difference in air quality in a filtered home. By reducing the amount of particles in your air, you also reduce the chances of spreading bacteria and viruses.

Cleanliness is Next to Godliness

Washing your hands is your number one protection against acquiring and spreading infectious disease. But you don't need to use antimicrobial soap to get the job done. It's been repeatedly shown that washing your hands with plain soap and water can kill germs that cause:

- The common cold

- Influenza

- Pneumonia

- Hepatitis A

- Acute gastroenteritis

- Stomach infections such as salmonella, campylobacter and norovirus

- Other contagious illnesses and surgical wound complications, including MRSA

According to *Becker's ASC Review,* scientists have found that various water temperatures had "no effect on transient or resident bacterial reduction." Not only does hot water not show any benefit, but it might increase the "irritant capacity" of some soaps, causing dermatitis. And using alcohol-based hand-hygiene products is in general no more effective than washing your hands with plain soap and water. In fact, contact dermatitis can develop from frequent and repeated use of hand hygiene products, exposure to chemicals and glove use.

Becker's also references a recent study comparing an antibacterial soap containing triclosan with a non-antibacterial soap. The results showed that the antibacterial soap did not provide any additional benefit. In addition, concerns have been raised about the use of triclosan because of the potential development of bacterial resistance.

However, it's important to use proper hand washing *technique.* To make sure you're actually removing the germs when you wash your hands, follow these guidelines:

1. Use warm water.

2. Use a mild soap.

3. Work up a good lather, all the way up to your wrists, for at least 20 seconds.

4. Make sure you cover all surfaces, including the backs of your hands, wrists, between your fingers, and around and below your fingernails.

5. Rinse thoroughly under running water.

6. Dry your hands with a clean towel or let them air dry.

7. In public places, use a paper towel to open the door as a protection from germs that the handles may harbor.

Also remember that your *skin* is actually your primary defense against bacteria, not the soap, so resist the urge to become obsessive about washing your hands. Over-washing can easily reduce the protective oils in your skin (especially in the winter and dry dessert environments) and cause your skin to crack—offering easy entry for bacteria and viruses into your body.

Instead, simply wash your hands when they look dirty, and prior to, or after, performing certain tasks that could spread infection.

- Before and after preparing food, especially when handling raw meat and poultry

- Before eating

- Before and after treating wounds or taking/giving medicine

- Before touching a sick or injured person

- Before inserting contact lenses

- After using the toilet or changing a diaper

- After touching an animal, its toys, leashes, or waste

- After blowing your nose or coughing/sneezing into your hands

- After handling garbage or potentially contaminated waste

Heavy Metal Contamination

Even when people follow healthy guidelines, they can still run into serious health problems.

One reason may be toxic metals. Mercury, aluminum, cadmium, arsenic, lead, nickel, and other metal poisons flood the environment and invade your body. Toxic metals can cause or contribute to a long list of diseases including Alzheimer's, Parkinson's, and other brain and neurological disorders. While the medical establishment recognizes the acute toxicity that comes from high levels of metals in your body, far more people suffer the adverse effects of low-level, chronic exposure.

Most of us need to detoxify our systems. The very first step in a detox program is to make sure you eat a healthy diet.

The next step is regular exercise. Make sure you sweat. Sweating excretes many toxins.

Drinking clean water also helps your body maintain its optimal state after you cleanse, as discussed in Chapter Five.

Do not start a detox if you are very sick. Otherwise, you can easily overwhelm your liver's ability to process the toxic substances that are being eliminated. That could make you even sicker. Start your healthy lifestyle *first,* before you detox, so you build a reserve for your body to draw on to let your liver do its job properly. The key is to not rely on cleansing as the detox. It's a great aid, but its benefits will be temporary, and it will be virtually useless unless you follow a good overall wellness program.

Then reduce your exposure to dangerous environmental metals in the first place by:

- using glass, cast iron, carbon steel, titanium, and enamel cookware.

- minimizing restaurant food.

- drinking from glass containers. Avoid plastic.

- not using cosmetics with aluminum bases, mineral powders that contain bismuth, and aluminum-laden antiperspirants.

- avoiding eating top of the food chain fish such as tuna.

- staying away from vaccinations containing mercury or aluminum.

- avoiding dental amalgam fillings.

- not drinking or bathing in unfiltered water.

When you see your anti-aging physician, make sure he or she orders you a urinalysis test for heavy metals, especially mercury and lead. If your levels are high, talk to your physician about the possibility of chelation therapy.

Chelation therapy has helped turn many people's lives around. In addition to flushing out toxic metals, it is often an effective alternative to bypass surgery.

However, either one is only a band-aid unless patients are willing to address the cause of their disease, which is usually, but not always, related to their diet and exercise.

Water and You

You can go a month without food but only a couple of days without water. It's the medium in which all your body's chemical reactions take place. It transports your nutrients, oxygen and waste products and regulates your body's temperature. Drinking enough pure water every day is one of the most ignored, most simple and cheapest ways to keep healthy.

Just how much water should you drink? When we're young, our bodies contain about 70% water. Once you pass forty, your hydration level is probably down to 60%. By age seventy, your levels are usually under 50%.

Contrary to popular belief, lean people are much more hydrated than the obese. And drinking water discourages rather than encourages water retention.

Even slight dehydration can disrupt critical cell functions. Studies have shown that people who drink eight or more glasses of water a day had less than one-fourth the risk of colon cancer than those who drank only two glasses a day. Water drinkers also get fewer headaches, muscle aches, hangovers, fatigue, constipation, heartburn, bladder and other cancers and valvular heart diseases.

To be properly hydrated, drink about one-half ounce of pure water a day for each pound of your body weight. If you weigh 160 pounds, that's ten 8-ounce glasses or a little less than seven 12-ounce glasses. Drink more if you exercise heavily or perspire heavily, and sip during the day for the most benefits rather than drinking a lot at once.

That doesn't mean soft drinks or energy drinks. If you want to age on the fast track, go right ahead. Just understand that food engineers would have a hard time designing more enticing dehydrating sugar-laden toxic potions. A 12-ounce can of Pepsi contains 10 teaspoons of sugar. Ten! And don't be lured into thinking the diet versions are better for you. They aren't.

As for the more popular energy drinks? Poison in a can. Take all the negative effects of soft drinks, then add enough caffeine to launch a rocket and you're begging for health problems way beyond the jitters and crashes your body endures.

Many municipal water utilities do not provide you with pure water. Water filtration systems have become very inexpensive and are well worth the cheap health insurance they provide for you. There are several sink top models available, but the healthiest water is produced by "selective filtration" products that have the ability to remove contaminants and not minerals. If you have a reverse osmosis unit, make sure you take a good mineral supplement. Some experts advocate water ionizers that alkalize your water.

The Sun

We discussed sun exposure in Chapter Seven when we talked about vitamin D3. The sun is a double-edged sword. Just the right amount is very healthful. Too much or too little isn't.

New research has discovered the counter-intuitive concept that going out in the sun at mid-day is best, not worst for your health.

Like most, I used to caution people to avoid the sun from 10:00 a.m. to 2:00 p.m. Well, it turns out that this is a case where a little bit of knowledge can actually be dangerous.

Cutaneous malignant melanoma (CMM) is the most serious form of skin cancer, accounting for about three-quarters of all skin cancer deaths. New studies now support that while avoiding the sun at mid-day will decrease your risk of painful sunburn, it will actually increase your cancer risk.

As it turns out, the optimal time to be in the sun for vitamin D production is actually between 10:00 a.m. to 2:00 p.m. The reason is two-fold.

First of all, you need a shorter exposure time because the UVB is more intense. The second reason is that when the sun gets lower in the sky, the UVB is filtered out much more than the UVA. And it turns out that the long wave of ultraviolet called UVA is highly correlated with melanoma—where the UVB is the one that produces vitamin D.

This surprising concept is just beginning to permeate through the mainstream media. For instance, the September 13, 2008, issue of *U.S. News & World Report* featured an article on time in the sun. In it, Robyn Lucas, an epidemiologist at Australian National University, agreed with these findings.

Both UVA and UVB can cause tanning and burning, although UVB tans and burns far more rapidly. UVA, however, penetrates your skin more deeply than UVB, and is thought to be a much more important factor in photoaging, wrinkles and skin cancers.

In Caucasian skin, twenty minutes of peak ultraviolet exposure may be optimal. It can take three to six times longer for darkly-pigmented skin to reach the equilibrium concentration of skin vitamin D. Longer exposures will be needed if sunbathing occurs at off-peak times for ultraviolet light or at the beginning or end of the summer. Gradually increase your time, starting in the spring. Aim toward exposing large areas of your skin to the sun.

So if you want to get out in the sun to maximize your vitamin D production, and minimize your risk of malignant melanoma, the middle of the day is the best and safest time to go. Just use a good natural sunscreen and/or protective clothing if you exceed these recommended exposure times.

Be cautious with prolonged exposure. One of the bigger factors in how old you look is how much sun you have been exposed to over the course of your lifetime. A suntan is actually a response by your skin cells to their DNA being damaged. Repeated, long-term exposure to direct sunlight has a direct effect on the appearance of your skin and could increase the likelihood that you will get skin cancer as you age. As a pre-emptive action, see a dermatologist every year or so to have every inch of your skin examined for cancer and other lesions.

If you have to be out in the sun for long periods, then find a good sun block with a very high SPF number. And make sure the block protects against both types of solar rays—UVA and UVB. Be aware that most commercial sun blocks can be toxic, and they screen out vitamin D3. Follow the recommendations in Chapter Seven for good sunscreen sources. If you take good antioxidants, including a 1:1 ratio of omega-3 and omega-6 oils, you will increase your resistance to skin damage from the sun.

If you want to live to your fullest potential, minimize the damage you do to your body on a daily basis. Take a good, hard look at the environment in which you spend your days, and see if you can eliminate frequent sources of molecular damage. You'll thank yourself in the long run!

Obesity

Most obesity is a direct result of lifestyle choices.

Obesity is becoming an epidemic. According to *National Health and Nutritional Surveys*, over the past ten years, the average woman's waistline has ballooned by almost two inches. They recorded higher blood sugar levels, and women aged 35–54 saw their incidence of strokes double over the same ten-year period.

Furthermore, as reported by the Centers for Disease Control and Prevention (CDC), in 1962, the average American woman was 5' 3" tall and weighed 120-125 pounds. In 2012, the average height was 5' 3.8", while the weight soared to 164.7 pounds. That shocked even me!

About one third of American adults are now obese, 70% are overweight, and it's getting worse every year. A fifty-two-year study tells us that, on average, obese people die seven years earlier than normal-weight adults. More recent studies show that the more people weigh, the older their cells appear on a molecular level, with obesity adding the equivalent of nearly nine years of age to a person's body! The study was led by St. Thomas Hospital in London.

In addition, obese people's brains look 16 years older than their healthy counterparts, and the overweight people's brains looked eight years older according to a new study published in Human Brain Mapping.

It also reports obese or overweight elderly people typically have significantly less brain tissue than normal weight people. The obese have 8% less on average, and those who are simply overweight have 4% less brain tissue.

According to a Surgeon General report, obesity is responsible for 300,000 deaths every year in the United States. From 1990 to 2000, obesity and inactivity-related deaths increased by 33%. Even more startling, according to the World Health Organization, 34% of the deaths in the world are linked to being overweight… and an astounding 71% in the United States.

And get this, researchers at Brigham and Women's Hospital in Boston determined that the risk for chronic diseases such as heart disease, colon cancer and diabetes is about TWENTY times higher for overweight people. Notice I did not say obese. It's even more deadly for them.

When's the last time you saw a really old fat person?

Why is obesity so deadly? Here are a few ways it affects your health:

- It raises your blood pressure.

- It causes type 2 diabetes. (The CDC tells us that one in four Americans is pre-diabetic or diabetic.)

- It triggers strokes as well as coronary disease, America's number one killer.

- It raises your risk of gallbladder disease.

- It increases your risk of many types of cancer. (Also according to the CDC, about one-third of all cancers are directly related to obesity.)

- It can cause metabolic syndrome, a cluster of killer medical conditions.

- It contributes to enlarged hearts, pulmonary embolism, ovarian cysts, gastro-esophageal reflux, fatty liver disease, hernias, erectile dysfunction, urinary incontinence, chronic renal failure, cellulitis, sleep apnea, osteoarthritis, gout and gallbladder disease/gall stones.

- It can lower your overall quality of life including poor body image, low self-esteem and depression.

The obese suffer 30–50% more health problems than problem drinkers—or even smokers.

So here are some tips:

Following Steps 1, 2 and 5 (Diet, Exercise and Lifestyle) will optimize your weight and extend your life and wellbeing. Obesity is a very big *risk*.

Some simple lifestyle basics are: move more, eat less and laugh every chance you get—especially at yourself.

And a good rule of thumb is, don't do the crazy things you did when you were eighteen.

Sleep

A UCLA Cousins Center research team reports that losing sleep for even part of one night can trigger the key cellular pathway that produces tissue-damaging inflammation. Your body perceives sleep deprivation as stress and responds by producing deadly stress chemicals. A single night of reduced sleep significantly impairs your ability to function. As you add days, impairment becomes cumulative.

This can become especially dangerous when driving or working around dangerous equipment or machinery. But it also increases mood swings, stress and irrationality; spikes your blood pressure; reduces your ability to adapt to change; impairs performance; saps your energy; slows reactions and impairs memory, judgment and decision making no matter what you do. Worse, you are often the last to notice or admit it. This has been clearly proven in clinical studies as well as in brain scans.

Even more alarming is, lack of sleep contributes to diabetes, obesity (through the work of a hormone called leptin that tells your brain when you're full), weakened immune system, depression, cancer, high blood pressure, heart disease and stroke. Also, a single night of sleeping just four, five or even six hours can impact your ability to think clearly. Sleep deprivation can cause changes in your brain activity similar to those experienced by people with psychiatric disorders. How many times have you deprived yourself of sleep by watching a television show that you forget about by the next day?

So lack of adequate sleep is definitely pro-aging. And if that's not enough reason to get enough quality sleep, consider the fact that sleep deprivation makes you a less active lover.

The average person needs seven to eight hours of *quality* sleep a night. Some need more, and some need less. If you're sick, under stress or pregnant, you may need more sleep. That means deep, undisturbed sleep. The darker you can make your room, the better. If you must get up in the middle of the night, do not turn on the light, if possible. And keep your bedroom quiet with little or no background noise or other interruptions.

Two good rules of thumb to follow are if you feel tired when you wake up, or if you frequently yawn throughout the day, you probably aren't getting enough sleep. Most of us have set times that we need to wake up in the morning, so getting more sleep, for most of us, means going to bed earlier. However, getting too much sleep may cause problems similar to not getting enough.

Helpful Hints for Deep, Rejuvenating Sleep:

Get regular exercise, but do not exercise shortly before going to bed.

➤ Adopt a regular sleep schedule. People who have a regular sleep schedule outperform those with erratic schedules, even though they get the same amount of sleep.

➤ Keep your TV out of your bedroom. It can tempt you to stay up late and can excite your mind when you want to relax.

➤ Go to bed earlier and get up earlier, rather than going to bed later and getting up later.

➤ If you drink coffee or tea, drink them early in the day.

➤ Reduce interruptive noise, even if you need to use some type of white noise machine. Heavy drapes can also reduce noise.

➤ Keep your bedroom as dark as possible.

➤ If you normally get up during the night to urinate, stop drinking liquids late in the day, and urinate right before bedtime.

➤ If you drink, do not have more than one or two alcoholic beverages in the evening. Excess alcohol disturbs your sleep cycle.

➤ Take a warm bath before bed.

➤ Keep your bedroom cool, under 70° F.

➢ Use a deep relaxation technique, or listen to a deep relaxation audio right before sleep.

➢ Quit working at least an hour before turning in to give your mind time to unwind.

➢ Supplement with: melatonin; sleep-inducing herbs such as kava, chamomile, valerian and/or ziziphus spinosa; 200–500 mg of calcium citrate; or 200–400 mgs of magnesium citrate right before bedtime.

One last word on sleep: What do you think about before falling asleep? Do you take your frustrations and anger to bed with you or do you think happy thoughts or think of your goals or problems you want solved? Your last thoughts before falling asleep are the ones your subconscious hears and works on during the night.

Longevity and Your Healthy Mouth

Did you know there is a strong correlation between the longevity of a person's teeth and their longevity in general?

Dental health can have wide-reaching effects on overall health. Poor oral health can make you susceptible to other health conditions.

A clean mouth contains several hundred billion bacteria, and this number increases tenfold when the mouth is not sufficiently cleaned.

Periodontitis is a chronic inflammatory oral disease that affects approximately 75% of U.S. adults. Periodontitis has harmful effects on overall wellness. It predisposes people to diabetes, insulin resistance, respiratory diseases, rheumatoid arthritis, obesity, osteoporosis, complications of pregnancy and cardiovascular diseases such as atherosclerosis, heart attack, congestive heart failure and coronary artery disease.

If you are planning to live a long time, it helps if you still have your own sound teeth. Poor dental health is as life shortening as smoking. Here are a few suggestions to care for your teeth and gums.

One of the best things you can do for the condition of your mouth is to gargle, or even better, WaterPik® with warm salt water. The salt water will kill many of the bacteria that inhabit your teeth and gums and will do a more effective job of removing and dissolving food debris than water alone.

Brushing and flossing are of course absolutely necessary for most of us but cannot always reach all the food particles in your mouth. That's why we suggest using a WaterPik® as part of your oral hygiene routine. Any bacteria you have in your mouth are there because they have a food source. A WaterPik® can remove nearly all the remaining food particles in your mouth.

Then finish the job with an Oral-B 500 electric toothbrush. It's the best I have found. And don't use detergent, commonly known as commercial toothpaste, on your teeth and gums, especially if you have red or swollen gums. Instead, rejuvenate your teeth and gums with Revitin Oral Therapy. You can find it at www.Revitin.com.

If you are really curious about how you are doing with your oral hygiene, you can buy plaque staining tablets at most pharmacies. The plaque will be temporarily dyed red on your teeth. Once you know where your problem areas are, you can focus on them better. But while brushing and flossing are important, they are not even close to the most important factor for healthy teeth. What is most important is your diet.

If you are already experiencing difficulties with your teeth or gums, we suggest you be wary of dentists who are overly eager to drill or perform root canals. Gum abscesses, for instance, are often mistaken for nerve abscesses, which require a root canal. Gum infections can be cured without any surgery, simply by your own aggressive steps, with good oral hygiene or by using antibiotics.

Even your regular dental checkup may be damaging to your teeth. When you have teeth scraped free of tartar, you assume a risk of scraping some of your enamel off as well. It is much more effective to simply dissolve away tartar than to scrape it.

It may also be untrue that you cannot regenerate your teeth if damage has occurred to them. You may be able to remineralize your teeth with a highly concentrated solution of calcium and phosphorus.

For more information on these subjects, look at Dr. Robert O. Nara's work. Dr. Nara founded an oral hygiene program called Oramedics. He wrote a book on the subject: *Money by the Mouthful: Everything That You Need to Know About the Health of your Mouth and Body That No Doctor's Going to Tell You.*

Finally, should you have your amalgam (silver) fillings removed? Some studies show they cause mercury poisoning from the mercury leeching from the fillings. Other studies show the levels of mercury are too low to cause harm, and that we are well-adapted to resisting mercury poisoning. It seems some people who are highly sensitive to mercury are the ones most affected, and some are seriously affected.

My recommendation is to never get amalgam fillings if you need your teeth filled. Opt for composites. It may be a good idea to have existing fillings replaced as long as they are removed properly. If not done correctly, removing them could release toxic amounts of mercury into your system. Learn about biomimetic dentistry. Research and interview dentists. If you're interested in progressive drill-free dentistry, you might first read Carol Vander Stoep's book, Mouth Matters.

Relationships

Are you in a loving relationship? Although some marriages could be detrimental to your health, married men typically live longer than single men. Part of the reason could be because women are more nurturing and make sure their men eat properly and take better care of themselves. But much of the added longevity stems from the psychological wellbeing of having a strong, loving relationship. Loneliness can shorten your life.

People with close friends, intimate relationships and loving pets are healthier, happier and live longer than those who don't. The more you stay connected, the longer you will live. If you're not in a happy relationship, fix or exit the one you have or find one. Close friendships contribute to longevity as well. You don't have to be married or even be in a love relationship to get some benefit.

But the most important relationship you can have is the one with yourself. Healthy positive thinking coupled with strong self-esteem will not only let you live longer and better but will make you want to live as long as possible. I recommend you buy a copy of *The Six Pillars of Self-Esteem* by Dr. Nathaniel Branden, and devour it.

Regular massage helps, too. Mutual massage between lovers is great for your health and your relationship, and therapeutic massage has tremendous benefits as well.

If you can't love a person, love a pet. Not only might people with pets live longer, but pets don't talk back or break up with you.

Finally, do you know you are the average of the five people you hang out with the most? Who you spend time with largely determines your state of health and longevity. If you associate with positive, upbeat, health-conscious people, their traits tend to rub off on you and give your wellbeing a boost. On the other hand, if your friends smoke, overeat, drink too much and have pessimistic outlooks on life, you probably won't live as long. This is yet another reason to teach your friends and family to be healthier.

When you're in the environment, you become the environment. You become those with whom you associate. So choose your friends carefully. If they resist your sound environment, the more you associate with them, the more likely you will be dragged down to their environment.

Here are two more ways to establish an environment conducive to optimal wellness and longevity.

First, clean up your kitchen. Snatch your life back from the purveyors of junk food. Never bring it into your home. Establish an environment at home that will enrich you rather than corrupt you. If you must eat junk food, do it somewhere else.

Second, step up your free time to support your health. Trade some of your mindless television and video game time that gets you fat and out of shape for time spent on exercise and education. Read books and articles on health. Watch educational videos or listen to CDs. Spend time with a personal trainer or nutritionist. Invest in yourself.

Maybe you're one of the lucky chosen few whose genetic makeup lets them get away with unhealthy habits. If you feel like rolling dice with your body, mind and your future, then go right ahead. But the vast majority will pay a heavy price for ignoring the advice you're getting here. Remember, your genes only account for about 25–35% of where you end up.

Most of those people adopt habits that cause tremendous damage to the old person they will soon become—slashing away years, or even decades, of vitality. This is a good example of time preference at work: we are hardwired to deeply discount the value of the future, even when it's our own future. What we don't value, we squander.

Without your health, you aren't capable of living a full life. Why squander it, now that you know better? Your good health today vastly increases your odds of capturing extreme youth and longevity. However, most of us slide gradually from youth, vitality and enthusiasm to deterioration and despair. A couple of decades of adding a few pounds here and there and gradually backing off on activity can transform you from the person you enjoyed being to faded looks, slipped performance and pessimism.

But here's good news. You have a second chance! Starting right now, today, you can get back almost 100% of what you lost. And when you succeed in living long enough to enjoy the fruits of radical life-extension technologies, you could be *better* than you were decades ago.

Your Personality Can Determine How Long You Will Live

"It's in their genes" is a common refrain from scientists when asked about factors that allow centenarians to reach age 100 and beyond. But researchers at Albert Einstein College of Medicine and Ferkauf Graduate School of Psychology of Yeshiva University have found that personality traits like being outgoing, optimistic, easygoing, and enjoying laughter as well as staying engaged in activities may also be part of the longevity genes mix. These findings were published online May 21, 2012 in the journal *Aging*.

More valuable insights regarding longevity predictors based on one's personality traits were uncovered in a famous eighty year study. You can find them all in *The Longevity Project: Surprising*

Discoveries for Health and Long Life from the landmark eight decade study by Howard S. Friedman and Leslie R. Martin.

They discovered the key predictor of long life is conscientiousness. Those who are persistent, well-organized, prudent, thrifty and responsible tend to live the longest.

You can change your personality if you want to. If you don't share most of the following life extending traits, you might consider adopting them:

- Stable and successful career

- Helping others and active in a large social network

- Heavy influence over your outcomes

- Non-critical, avoid arguments and don't always try to get things your own way

- Not reactionary with hostility to personal slights

- Motivated

- Engaged in personal goals

- Look for good in people

- Work and family are important

- Choose your work rather than being thrown into it

Show Me the Money

Monitoring stock market uncertainties made one thing crystal clear to me. You may need money if you want to dodge the grim reaper. Lots of it. If you didn't lose money in 2008, it might be because you didn't have any to lose. And yes, that could be bad if you want to live for an extremely long time.

Let's face it. The first people who are going to get effective life extending treatment are those who will be able to afford it. If you're old and broke when the longevity boat arrives, you might miss it. Sure, prices will come down, and pretty rapidly too. But many of us are on the bubble as it is, and not being near the front of the line could just cost you your life. So what are you going to do about it?

All your life, you have been told to save for the future, and you're most certainly familiar with the magic of compound interest. As we age, we may regret not having started saving years ago. Now, many people who didn't save believe it's too late to amass any kind of fortune, so they live day-to-day, paycheck-to-paycheck. But what if you knew beyond a shadow of a doubt, you would be biologically transformed into a 25-year old, twenty or thirty years from now, if you had $500,000 in the bank at that time. Do you realize socking away $30,000 in a segregated investment account that compounded at around 10% growth per year, would give you your $500,000 in less than thirty years? (10% is roughly the historical annual growth of the stock market.)

In other words, $30,000 could be the difference between your being part of the last generation to die from aging... or part of the first generation to live endlessly. What if you don't have $30,000? That's easy. Save $3,000 now and $3,000 every year in the same type of account, and presto! You'll have your magical $500,000 in less than thirty years.

I have no idea what full rejuvenation will cost when it's available, so plan for more, not less. When planning, factor in inflation.

The insidious hidden tax called inflation continually erodes your wealth. Although U.S inflation rates over the past twenty years averaged 2.5%, medical care's rate of inflation has currently been running about 1% higher than inflation on all goods and services. Over the past ten years, inflation devoured 28% of your overall buying power, medical care increased by 47%, and hospital and related services ballooned by 86% (U.S. Department of Labor: Bureau of Labor Statistics). So plan accordingly. If you err on the high side and save too much, won't it be nice to be young again with a pile of money in the bank?

Disaster Insurance

Now that you see how important financial solvency could be to your survival and how fragile our economy can be, what are even more fragile are developed country societies in general. Most of us depend heavily on the grid. But what happens when the grid fails? Entire neighborhoods, cities or even regions can go down.

For the most part, we are extremely dependent. A simple interruption in the grid could put a sudden break in your supply of food, water, fuel and power and access to medical care, clothing and supplies. And what could break the grid? Any number of things actually. They could include but not be limited to: hurricanes, floods, earthquakes, fires, tornadoes, war, terrorism (nuclear, biological, chemical, etc), social unrest caused by poor economic times or by any of the preceding upheavals.

Even a few days' interruption in food supplies could cause wide-scale rioting and plundering. And social unrest could endanger your life.

This is nothing new to you, but I'll bet you don't think much about it, do you?

I'm optimistic, yet I understand the harsh realities of the frailty of modern civilization. Given enough time, the chances are you will be affected by at least one of these life-threatening events. So if you truly cherish life and plan on living for a long time, wouldn't it be prudent to insure yourself against disasters?

Your best insurance is self-reliance. That could mean any or all of the following:

➢ Installing a security system in your home

➢ Storing a minimum of 30 days' supply of food and water, candles, flashlights, batteries, antibiotics, a first aid kit, firearms, a propane/kerosene heater, survival books, air filters/masks, radiation pills and portable wealth such as cash, gold and silver coins and maybe even diamonds

➢ Installing a generator and a water filter in your home

➢ Living in a safe neighborhood, community or region

➢ Living a fairly low-profile life unless you can afford to live in a secure compound. Avoid being easy prey or a tempting target.

Yes, I know, I sound like a "doom and gloomer." The fact is I'm a long-term optimist but a short-term pessimist who knows anything can go wrong at any time. Doesn't it make sense to protect what could be your open-ended life?

Who's in Charge?

We work overtime to make extreme life extension a reality for you. But we fight an ongoing battle with a deadly enemy only you have control over.

That enemy is your personal lifestyle.

Since it may be touch and go whether or not we can reverse aging in your lifetime, how long you keep yourself alive can be the difference between oblivion and open-ended youth. We're doing all we can to push you over the finish line. Are you doing the same for yourself?

Remember, *you* are the one with most of the power over your destiny. It's not your genes. It's not your environment. It's you!

By now, you understand your lifestyle can be the difference of up to twenty extra or twenty fewer years. You should also know what you can do to add (or subtract) those years, especially after you finish reading *Smart, Strong and Sexy at 100?*

So what are you doing about it? Are you focusing on the benefits you will receive? Or are you giving in to deadly short-term habitual temptations?

Stop right now, and do this exercise. Consider the things that are keeping you from being as fit as you can be. What are those things you could change if you had a magic wand? You might want to stop and list them on a piece of paper.

Then go back in time to the first time you noticed those destructive habits creeping into your life. Step into your body at that time and feel the pain they have caused you. Now gradually bring yourself back to the present and review the pain, regret and even sickness they have caused you at each phase of your life. Consider how they have affected your wellness, appearance, self-esteem, relationships and career. Now fast forward to the future and observe how they will continue to eat away at your happiness, shorten your life *and cause you to miss out on endless youth.*

Feel the pain and loss these habits will cause if you don't change them. Consider the lost hope and the unfulfilled dreams.

Now come back and realize that you are the one with the ability to seize control of your life, your body and mind, your long future and your happiness.

So who's in charge? If not you, then consider the words of Ayn Rand.

"...if you choose to perish, do so with full knowledge of how cheaply so small an enemy has claimed your life."

Now that you know what to do, read on to see how to keep it all from unwinding.

CHAPTER 10. STEP 6—STRESS MANAGEMENT

Stress drains you from the inside, robbing your energy and vitality. Stress speeds up the aging process, leads to fatigue and will silently sabotage even the strongest motivation. Do everything right—everything—and chronic stress can crash it all down!

Even a few minutes of focused stress reduction every day is a powerful way to prevent disease and accelerate your regeneration.

I'm going to show you how to not only reduce your chronic stress, but also how to avoid most of it.

Just like exercise, emotion signals your cells to grow strong or weak. The same molecular pathways go to work for you or against you. Stress, hostility and loneliness starve your cells and put them in danger. However, optimism and love trigger growth. Like deciding to exercise, you can pretty much master your emotions. It's a choice.

Consider this: Real Age reports that people who feel more stressed have telomeres that are almost 50% shorter than those of people who say they are less stressed. This equates to a whopping nine to seventeen-year difference in biological age!

How much stress do you experience during the average day? Chronic stress kills, you know. It kills by: weakening your immune system; disrupting your digestive system; causing heart disease, stroke, cancer, Alzheimer's and more. In fact, the U.S. National Academy of Sciences estimates that 70 to 80% of all family doctor visits are stress-related. And leading medical authorities estimate that 90% of all diseases are caused or complicated by stress. This was reported by the Congressional Prevention Coalition.

In addition to the above, these conditions include high blood pressure, kidney damage, ulcers, food allergies, diabetes and obesity. Cortisol, the main stress hormone, even causes your lean muscle to break down while increasing the storage of fat. Want to be a lean energy machine? Then learn to relax.

Stress can affect every one of the trillions of cells in your body. In essence, chronic stress accelerates aging and makes you sick. Why do everything else right, only to lose it all to stress?

What Causes Stress?

I have concluded there is one overriding cause of stress. In fact, it may be the only cause. In one word, it's "reaction."

Reaction to workplace pressures is the most common source of stress. Gallup reports 80% of employees suffer from stress. And stressed-out employees suffer from two to three times as much work injury as their non-stressed counterparts.

Most stress is caused by changes in your life and the sense of being out of control. Being out of control is usually caused by being in this reactionary mode, letting external events or other people control your actions, rather than your actions determining the external events in your life. Most of us feel stressed much of the time due to these two factors.

Some ways around this are to monitor and list all your daily events. Then decide which ones are truly important to you and which aren't. Then act on those that are important.

Do you tend to react to things that seem urgent at the expense of ignoring or procrastinating on those that are important? Your key is purposeful action and avoiding procrastination. When you procrastinate, your events control you.

You probably know what thoughts and actions advance you forward in life. I trust you know what specific action or actions energize you and are most productive for you. What are you best at? What do you enjoy doing? Know these answers. Focus on those related activities, and you will cut 90% of the stress out of your life. In other words, get "proactive." Take control of your life one day at a time.

Is that how you manage most of your average day? Probably not. If you do, congratulations! But if you're like me, you're constantly faced with interruptions and distractions: phone calls, emails, family emergencies, arguments, mail, traffic jams, unexpected guests, financial problems, tax issues, bill paying, other peoples' agendas, etc, etc, etc.

Chronic stress is often these continual minor stressors over an extended period of time. The cumulative effect slowly erodes your body over time at your cellular level if you don't make a conscious effort to let your body recover.

Managing Stress

So how do you keep this insidious killer from robbing you of your health, happiness and prosperity? It's actually very simple. Plan your days in advance. Fill your schedule with positive uplifting actions that move you toward your goals. Go back a few weeks in your calendar, and list all your counterproductive reactionary items. Do the same moving forward for the next two weeks. Every time you react to something, and every time you feel stress, write it down. Write down what you hate doing as well.

Then group these items and hand them off. Delegate them. Outsource them. Or just ignore the ones that won't damage you if they don't get done.

Second, work in peace, quiet and privacy. Shut distractions out during designated chunks of your work day. Turn off your phone and email during these periods. Close your door, and leave specific instructions to not bother you except in extreme emergencies such as a medical crisis or anything else that is absolutely life, family or business threatening. Start in small steps and work your way up until you completely control most of your work day.

Once you master these habits, you'll wonder why you didn't do so years ago. Your business and personal life will prosper like never before. And you'll live longer.

(By the way, I was interrupted twice while writing this section, because I am not behind a closed door. Being distracted and then trying to refocus doubled the time it should have taken me to write this. I'm writing this book to myself as much as to you. So I need to keep reminding myself, over and over. The rewards far outweigh the effort.)

Even productive living creates stressful situations. As long as you're in action, you will always have some stress in your life. Self-imposed deadlines, major changes in your life and others can create stress.

We simply don't grow without stress. Some stress is good for you. It evolved as a survival mechanism. Without it, we don't adapt and become strong. It gives you a rush of adrenalin when you're faced with a sudden life-threatening situation. You react faster, often without even thinking. Your strength can suddenly double for an instant.

What kills you is not adapting to the chronic stresses of life. Now that we're civilized (at least technologically), we seldom face life-threatening events (unless you live in Detroit). However, modern life puts other pressures on you. Instead of being attacked by a wild animal, escaping and then relaxing for a week, we get stressed by the multiple processes of living in a complex world. And this stress doesn't end as fast as it occurred. Stressful situations may stay with us for days, weeks and even years. Or they may pop up one after another. They can make us feel as helpless as babies. Sometimes they spin our lives out of control. They all cause our stress system to activate. The system designed to help us in an emergency becomes dangerous to our health if it runs all the time.

Physical and emotional stress causes the release of cortisol and catecholamines (adrenaline and noradrenaline), hormones that keep the body performing under high stress situations. As I mentioned, these hormones are good in short bursts, such as in emergency situations, but damaging after long periods of exposure.

Catecholamines are also known as the "fight or flight" hormones, because they "rev up" your system (increase blood pressure and heart rate) in response to stress. Cortisol suppresses normal inflammatory responses and immune functions to allow you to continue to perform in an emergency. Long-term exposure to cortisol and catecholamines, however, is linked to a whole host of physiological problems, including memory loss, immune system inhibition, endocrine system disruption, increased free radical production, chronic increased blood pressure and chronic increased heart rate.

This chronic stress is what kills us instead of saving us. So we need to make stress reduction and relaxation a priority in our lives if our plans are peace, health and longevity. The good news is it's not hard to do.

All you need to do is stop and get off the horse once in a while. Relaxation is not only fun and easy, but it will extend your life and help keep you from getting sick.

Focus and intentional practice are much more effective than passive relaxation. You might practice meditation, yoga, prayer, self-hypnosis, deep breathing exercises, creative visualization, listening to soothing sounds such as nature sounds or relaxing music, soaking in a tub, biofeedback and tai chi.

There are many other stress busters out there. The more stress management tools you learn and use regularly, the happier and healthier you'll be. Stress management can measurably reverse much of the stress-induced damage very quickly. You can even restore over-taxed immune systems in ninety days or less. Best of all, your benefits accumulate. The longer you practice stress management techniques, the healthier you become.

You are responsible for much of the emotional stress placed on your body. If you perceive a situation as stressful, your body will react. If you can manage difficult situations without overreacting, you save your body from unnecessary chemical damage.

Drs. T. H. Holmes and R. H. Rahe researched the strong correlation between stressful situations and illness. Then they devised a *Social Readjustment Scale.*

To see whether you are in danger of illness, look at the chart below, and add up the number of Life Crisis Units (LCUs) you have received in the past two years. If you are in danger, take immediate steps to alleviate your stress and return to a more healthy condition. For example, one-time cardiac patients who learned to manage their stress reduced their heart attack/heart problem risk by an incredible 74%.

LCUs	Probability of Illness
300	80%+
200–299	50%
150–199	33%

EVENT	LCUs	EVENT	LCUs
Death of spouse	100	Son or daughter leaving home	29
Divorce	73	Trouble with in-laws	29
Separation	65	Outstanding personal	
Jail term	63	achievement	28
Death of close		Spouse begins or stops work	26
family member	63	Begin or end of school or college	26
Personal illness or injury	53	Change in living conditions	25
Marriage	50	Change in personal habits	24
Fired at work	47	Trouble with boss	23
Marital reconciliation	45	Change in work	
Retirement	45	hours or conditions	20
Change in health		Change in residence	20
of family member	44	Change in school or college	20
Pregnancy	40	Change in recreation	19
Sex difficulties	39	Change in church activities	19
Gain of new family member	39	Change in social activities	18
Business readjustment	38	A moderate loan or mortgage	17
Change in financial state	38	Change in sleeping habits	16
Death of close friend	37	Change in number of	
Change to a different		family get-togethers	15
line of work	36	Change in eating habits	15
Change in number		Holiday	13
of arguments with spouse	35	Christmas	12
A large mortgage or loan	30	Minor violations of the law	11
Foreclosure of			
mortgage or loan	30		

Of the several things you can do to control your stress and lessen its detrimental effects, one of the first is to eliminate any artificial chemical stress you might be putting on your body. Your body has a hard enough time managing stress without its stress management system turned on by external chemicals.

Although a little caffeine may have healthy attributes, it also releases excess cortisol and catecholamines. So it mimics the effect of stress. High blood sugar, caused by consuming high levels of carbohydrates (especially food high in refined sugar) can also mimic the effects of stress by causing large doses of insulin to be released into your blood stream. High insulin levels then cause release of cortisol, suppressing your immune system. Salt is one other chemical stressor, because it can unnaturally raise your blood pressure.

Previous Longevity Express Steps

Taking care of your body goes a long way towards helping you cope with these situations. The nutrition, exercise and supplementation routines mentioned in steps 1, 2 and 3 will better equip you to deal with the stresses placed on your body. A good diet and supplements help you cope with increased production of free radicals caused by stress. Exercise reduces stress and increases your cardiovascular ability to handle stress while increasing your antioxidant potential. Do you notice how often exercise keeps popping up? Exercise and diet are paramount. If you don't like exercise, at least go out for regular brisk walks.

In addition, when faced with difficult situations, make sure you get enough rest. Fatigue can definitely reduce your immune function and healing ability.

Besides exercise, many physical relaxation techniques can manage the effects of your stress. A stress management relaxation technique designed by the Institute of HeartMath has raised DHEA (your master hormone) levels by 100% and reduced the stress hormone cortisol by 23% in just one month.

We're basically descended from nervous monkeys with hair-trigger fight-or-flight responses. The region of your brain that processes fear can override the rest of your brain's ability to think logically. So you need to learn to relax. Some of the best techniques are meditation and deep breathing. Did you ever notice how fast and shallow you breathe when you are stressed? It's hard to breathe deeply and feel anxious or tense at the same time. Try it.

Meditation doesn't just have to be for eastern mystics. Millions of Americans practice it, because its health benefits have been proven in many different studies. It's not an escape, as some think. Meditation is a proactive practice that can enhance your life. It's the equivalent of giving your mind an escape valve to blow off steam.

All meditation really means is to focus on one thing for an extended period of time. This allows your mind to reset itself and stop the vicious cycle of thinking about things that stress you out.

Focus separates peak performers from average performers, possibly more than any other attribute. It also builds energy. That's why so many high profile leaders practice meditation. Meditation is anything that brings you to the moment and keeps you there. The more you meditate and focus on the "now," the stronger you grow physically, mentally and emotionally.

Mainstream medicine is now beginning to take notice of meditation's effects. For example, mindfulness-based cognitive therapy (MBCT), which is about 80% meditation, has been approved in Britain for use with people who have experienced three or more episodes of depression.

Your brain, just like your muscles, can be overworked, and it needs recovery time. Like many people who exercise, meditators in their mid-fifties evaluated by Dr. Robert Keith Wallace tested twelve years biologically younger than non-meditators. Did you know meditation actually increases the thickness of your brain regions associated with attention and sensory processing? Here are some additional benefits:

Meditating…

➢ increases the growth of new brain cells.

➢ increases your IQ and Emotional Intelligence scores.

➢ increases your comprehension and productivity.

➢ improves your mental focus, memory and decision making.

➢ decreases stress, anxiety and depression.

➢ reduces free radicals, heart rate and biological aging.

➢ slows your breathing.

➢ improves quality of and ability to sleep.

➢ reduces your blood pressure.

➢ relaxes your muscles.

➢ reduces your risk of stroke or heart attack.

➢ gives your body time to eliminate lactic acid and other waste products.

➢ increases blood levels of DHEA.

➢ reduces anxiety and eliminates stressful thoughts.

➢ helps with clear thinking.

➢ helps with focus and concentration.

➢ reduces irritability.

➢ accelerates weight loss.

➢ reduces stress headaches.

➢ enhances overall health.

Wow! Is that incredible, or what? Review this list a few times. Let the benefits sink in. Who wouldn't want better health, to think more clearly, to age more slowly and to be smarter?

The essence of meditation is to quiet your thoughts by focusing completely on just one thing. Unlike hypnosis, which is more of a passive experience, meditation is an active process that seeks to exclude outside distractions by concentrating all your thoughts on the subject of meditation.

In all cases, it helps if your body is relaxed. Get in a position that you can comfortably sustain for a period of time (20–30 minutes is ideal, but even five minutes helps a lot). If you choose, and if you are sufficiently supple, the lotus position may work best for you. Otherwise, sitting in a comfortable chair or lying on a bed may be equally effective.

A number of different focuses of concentration may be used. Which one you choose is a matter of personal taste. Some of these are detailed below:

> *Breathing:* Focus on each breath in and out, breathing in through your nose on a count of seven, hold for a count of three, and breathe out through your mouth on a count of eight. Inhale and exhale completely, totally filling and emptying your lungs.

> *Focusing on an object:* Completely focus on one object. Choose something pleasant and interesting, and then examine it in detail. Observe its color, shape, texture, etc.

> *Focus on a sound:* Some people like to focus on sounds. The classic example is the Sanskrit word "Om," meaning "perfection."

> *Imagery:* Create a mental image of a pleasant and relaxing place in your mind. Involve all your senses in the imagery: see the place, hear the sounds, smell the aromas, feel the temperature and the wind.

In all cases, keep your attention focused. If external thoughts or distractions wander in, let them drift out. If necessary, visualize attaching the thoughts to objects and then move the objects out of your attention.

Now I'm going to show you two simple stress-busting techniques that work like crazy with minimal time and effort. In fact, they are fun. They'll take you from a dysfunctional, tied-up-in-a-bundle-of-knots condition to the relaxed, happy and productive super-star you are meant to be in a matter of minutes.

Deep Breathing

It's fun and easy. It's also a proven technique that has worked for thousands of years in virtually every culture in history.

Simply sit or lie in a comfortable position. Close your eyes, briefly clear your mind, and take a slow, deep, belly breath through your nose. Then exhale slowly through your mouth. Repeat while focusing only on your breath. If other thoughts enter your mind, simply let them pass through, and keep focusing on your breath.

When I first tried this, I had a hard time focusing on, or visualizing, my breath. After some trial and error, I came up with a way that works—at least for me.

I visualize the healing air I breathe in as gold and silver, relaxing, recharging molecules or particles, representing all the peace, tranquility and goodness in the world. I see the exhaled air as smoky pollution… cleansing my body of toxins and stress.

I do this several times a day. To demonstrate how effective this simple technique can be, I did it last evening when I felt stress over an unpleasant task. When I started, my blood pressure was 117/75. Seven minutes later, I dropped it to 97/63. That's simply amazing! Had I not taken my stress break, I would have eroded my health, functioning sub-par and frenzied. Instead, I jumped back into my task with renewed energy and motivation.

This is not a one-time event. I get these results regularly. Taking several stress-busting breaks every day could help you avoid 80% of all medical conditions. That's the medical profession's conservative estimate of the toll stress takes on you.

How often do you think what you are doing is so urgent and important that you can't afford to take one minute off, let alone seven? Well, I've got news for you. The best time to take a stress break is when you think you don't have the time. That's exactly when proactive relaxation breaks are the most productive way to spend your time. Not only will they improve your performance, but you could avoid a nasty hospital stay, or even a premature death as a side effect.

Release Your Tension

Do you ever hurt from muscle tension? Dr. Neil Fiore offers a 5-minute and 39-second solution. I have an outline below, but even better, go to www.neilfiore.com to download a free MP3 file that walks you through it.

Feeling tense now? Then try the following to loosen up.

Dr. Fiore's tension busting steps:

1. Sit up straight with your feet on the floor.
2. Notice your body, head to toe, starting at your scalp, to your jaw, neck, shoulders and so forth, down to your feet.
3. Notice any areas of tension.
4. Inhale fully, and hold your breath.
5. Tighten all your muscles, clench your fists, lift your feet from the floor and press them together, and suck in your belly.
6. Exhale and release completely, letting all your muscles relax.
7. Repeat several times.

There it is. It's much easier to relax tense muscles by tightening them fully first than by just trying to relax them. The secret? Tension to relaxation by exhaling. Now download Dr. Fiore's audio.

What Else Can You Do?

In addition to the suggestions above, I recommend looking into how well you manage your life. One of the primary causes of stress is the feeling of being out of control. Techniques such as personal goal setting and time management can help you feel like you have a better handle on your life. Also, simplify your life as much as possible. Complexity is a major contributor to damaging stress.

Other stress reducers include supplementing with DHEA. Lowering your stress hormones usually results in higher levels of

DHEA. A majority of depressed patients show depressed DHEA levels. There is also evidence that chronic stress lowers your blood levels of omega-3s, so make sure you are supplementing with high-quality fish oil if you are stressed.

Ingest certain herbs like green tea (use the matcha version) or chamomile, skullcap, valerian, lemon balm and lavender; eat a wide variety of fresh fruits and vegetables; get enough quality sleep; exercise; take regular vacations, and take regular breaks during the work day. During your breaks, do deep-breathing exercises, eat a small snack or meal, work out—and most of all, completely detach from your work and any problems.

Many people see an immediate improvement in their stress after a spinal adjustment. That's because stress usually causes you to chronically tense your upper back and shoulder region. That often causes your vertebrae to misalign.

Loneliness or horrible relationships can stress you to death as well. On the other hand, loving relationships can be calming and health-promoting. Couples who had physical contact, such as a brief hug and ten minutes of hand-holding, actually lowered their heart rates and blood pressure by up to 50%, according to researchers at the University of North Carolina-Chapel Hill. And a previous study determined that hugging and hand-holding reduce the negative effects of stress.

Group relationships can be as important as relationships with a loved one. A deep sense of relationship with your community, whether religious, ethnic or even geographic, can lower your risk of heart attack or cancer.

And once you shift your relationship with time, from a frenzied time-is-running-out consciousness to a more relaxed approach, you'll notice a calming stress-free effect that opens you up to healing, happiness and increased productivity. Once you start your personal longevity program, you'll begin to realize your productive, healthy years don't have to be crammed into sixty years or less. Extending them through your eighties and way beyond will liberate you to take a more relaxed and healthier approach to your life and career.

Unfortunately, the old wives' tale about stress turning your hair gray is in many respects true. Because of the damage to multiple systems in your body, people who are constantly exposed to stress are much more likely to appear and feel older. So use all these techniques to your advantage, and maintain your youth.

How about retirement? Do you think that would be a stress reducer? Think again. Studies show that on average, people who retire die earlier than those who continue working. Does that mean you should never retire from your job or business? No. Retiring from your job is fine. But if you want a long and healthy life, never retire from meaningful activities. Get involved with mentoring younger generations or with charities, for example. Golf and fishing aren't considered "meaningful activities."

You'll notice the emphasis on "managing" your stress rather than avoiding it. We can't avoid change, and change can certainly cause stress. Change and stressful situations can bring you loads of enjoyment. They can heighten your experiences; intensify relationships, love and joy; maximize creativity and draw out your passion and vitality. You can often transform your stress into positive emotions.

Sitting in a cave, hiding from the world, might bring some tranquility, but there's something to be said for participating in the enormous amount of adventures and opportunities available to you. Without an active role, and without change and variety, long life could prove to be meaningless.

The Lifehack.org website gives us some more simple tips.

➢ **Make quiet time:** Whether you meditate daily or just spend an hour a night with a book, you need to create a space where you can clear your mind.

➢ **Eat better:** A good diet can help your body better deal with the effects of stress.

➢ **Make family time:** Eat at least one meal a day with your family (or with friends if you're single).

➢ **Talk it out:** Bottling up your frustrations, even the little ones, leads to stress.

➢ **Prioritize:** Figure out what in your life actually needs attention and what doesn't.

➢ **Accept interruptions gracefully:** Leave enough wiggle room so you can adapt to changes in your day.

➢ **Pay attention to yourself:** Notice when you feel stressed, and determine the cause.

➢ **Love:** Build relationships. Share yourself. Feel human warmth.

Finally, Some Words of Wisdom on Stress from Author, Philosopher and Entrepreneur Robert Ringer:

> Consider that children, jobs, lack of time, and other frazzling issues that most of us have to deal with are not the underlying causes of stress. Rather, stress is a self-imposed mental state. Stress is opposite of serenity. So strive for peace of mind, because you cannot simultaneously experience tranquility and stress.
>
> Fear, loneliness, rejection, illness, death, financial failure, and loss of love are just a few examples of the kinds of sadness and misfortune we all have to deal with from time to time. Where we differ is how we handle them.
>
> The foundation is "living right." That means always being conscious of, and vigilant about, making good choices. But I'll bet you've had times where you did something that, in your gut, didn't feel right. And just as many experiences where you did not do something that you knew, deep down inside, you should have done.
>
> In fact, you can apply the "feels right/feels wrong" barometer to virtually any aspect of life. Whenever a person who's a hundred pounds overweight walks by me at a ballpark—beer in one hand and container of gooey, cheese-covered nachos in the other—I think to myself, "Surely this gal must know that what she's doing is not in her best interest."
>
> Specifically, she knows that it's wrong for her health and longevity, but in reality, she doesn't think about it in such specific

terms. Her stress level simply rises and brings with it a higher level of unhappiness.

Or how about when you do something that, at the deepest level of your moral foundation, doesn't feel honest? This often brings guilt into your life and stress.

Know thyself.

The real key to conquering stress is self-examination—continual, honest self-examination regarding the harmony and disharmony in your life. Inner conflict causes stress. How many times has a lingering personal conflict squeezed your chest and tied your stomach in a knot? That's chronic stress in action. For maximum health and longevity, release those pent up emotions and settle your conflicts immediately.

In contrast to conflict, leading a concentric life (i.e., one in which what you do matches up closely with what you believe in and what you say) brings harmony into your world.

Shake the habit of fretting and stewing about problems that don't exist.

It's amazing how many people live in a "what if" world. Projecting medical problems is an excellent and all-too-common example. Medical students are notorious for imagining they've contracted some terrible disease. The reason, of course, is they study diseases on a daily basis.

Can there be a better definition of joy than the feeling you have when the results of your prostate exam, colonoscopy, pap smear, or mammogram come back negative? Until you get that thumbs-up feedback from your doctor or lab, it's very easy for your mind to play tricks on you and stress you to the limit.

If you excessively dwell on bad things that might happen in your life—medical or otherwise—you only succeed in increasing the chances of their actually happening. Focus on today's problems, because, in most cases, that's a full-time job.

Recognize that for every negative, there's an offsetting positive.

The universe is in balance. For every positive, there's an offsetting negative, and for every negative, there's an offsetting positive. Balance is the natural order of the universe.

The nice thing about it is that when you understand and believe in universal balance, it gives you the mind-set to look quickly and automatically for the offsetting positive in every negative situation.

Accept the inevitable.

Notwithstanding the Natural Law of Balance, there are some things you simply can't do anything about. However, it's important to be able to discern the difference between inevitable and difficult. For example, success can be difficult, but, regardless of one's circumstances, failure is not inevitable. Accepting the inevitable is not being negative, it's actually positive. What's negative is not being able to ignore the inevitable and move on with your life.

Accepting the inevitable and focusing on opportunities in your life is virtually guaranteed to lower your stress level.

Refuse to react to the negative remarks disseminated by others.

Just don't make the naive mistake of expecting everyone to love you, because they won't. Remember, even Mahatma Gandhi was assassinated.

Intellectualize the reality that life isn't perfect.

Just about everyone claims to understand this reality, but I don't believe most people take the trouble to analyze what it really means. One of the most traumatic moments of children's lives is when they discover their parents aren't perfect. Likewise, I believe that one of the most traumatic moments of a parent's life is when he/she discovers that his/her child isn't perfect. You can reduce your stress many times over by accepting the reality that there is no perfect child, parent, spouse, home, city, or job.

I'm going to share with you two anti-stress techniques that can be very difficult to master. Even so, I can assure you that it will be worth your while to do, because I don't believe a low stress level and peace of mind are possible without them.

Don't try to make the world bend to your will.

Trying to get everyone to do things your way goes beyond stress. It's a frustrating, hopeless exercise that can drive a person mad. This is an area where you have to be careful, even when dealing with your own children. While it's a parent's responsibility to teach and guide his/her children, the wise parent learns early on that they cannot and will not do everything exactly as their parents want them to. The reality is that your children are different human beings than you, so it would be unnatural for them to mirror you 100% of the time.

Control anger and bitterness.

It's worth repeating Ralph Waldo Emerson's famous words: "For every minute you are angry, you lose sixty seconds of happiness."

I remember a friend once telling me about a guy who had shafted him out of a lot of money. I asked how he could be so calm about it, and I'll never forget his response: "I've found that it's disarming to just smile, be polite, and act as though nothing is wrong. Not only do you avoid making enemies by handling things in this manner, you also save yourself a ton of aggravation. All you need to do is avoid having business dealings with that person in the future. And to the extent you are cordial, he'll probably even sing your praises to everyone— which means you win all the way around."

Whenever I become angry, I give myself time to cool off before saying or doing something that I might later regret.

Robert Ringer publishes an excellent free newsletter called *A Voice of Sanity in an Insane World.* You can subscribe to it at www. robertringer.com.

So as you can see, it's not events that shape your world. It's your thought processes. Your mental state will always be the most important factor when it comes to achieving peace of mind. Here's a proactive event that will improve your mental state: Relaxation. Is it proactive? Yes. Purposely relaxing actually accomplishes a lot. It rests and rejuvenates your mind and your body. The bottom line is, relaxed people are healthier, happier, more productive and live longer—much longer.

I have more to say about thought processes and how to supercharge your happiness and health in the next chapter on the final step, #7, Attitude.

But before I let you escape from this topic, here are some of musings on stress from one of the most fun guys I know and a true Renaissance man, John Carlton:

The first rule for battling stress—if you can't walk away from it (which is actually the best rule, when you can pull it off)—is to be healthy. Because stress destroys everything good in your system... and uncorks massive floods of the bad stuff. Your endorphins get smothered and gang-raped by adrenaline and stomach acid.

For example: I love me some hamburgers. Yes, I do. So once a month (sometimes twice) I treat myself to a burger-and-fry orgy at In-And-Out.

Not every day. Not every week.

Every once in a while.

I've got friends who are fit and thin, subsisting on twigs and lawn clippings, who never, ever, ever, ever even *think* about eating a slice of pizza.

Okay, they're happy (or smug) about being healthy. But no pizza, ever? That's not enjoying a successful life in my book.

Still, life is for living. Passion, desire, and raw urges are part of the deal... as long as you maintain moderation according to your system. (That means, some of you can't indulge in some things, because you can't moderate it. So you don't do those things, or drink that stuff, or subject yourself to situations where you lose all sense of moderation.)

Stress loves it when you go overboard, on anything. Work, romance, sports, hobbies, day trading, video games, whatever. We're an obsessive species, for sure.

That still doesn't mean you have to live like a monk.

Wanna know a secret? I've hung out with athletes, trainers, health guru's, doctors and other health-oriented experts for decades...

... and most of them do NOT live a strict life of no-fun.

The really successful ones have... wait for it... mastered the art of MODERATION.

Newest Findings

Now that I've devoted an entire chapter to how bad stress is for you, and how to manage it, I'm going to eat some of my words. We're constantly learning, and at an ever increasing rate. Here's some surprising new information that sheds a different light on stress:

Two studies suggest your *attitude* toward stress may be a bigger health risk than the stress itself. A 2012 University of Wisconsin-Madison School and Medicine and Public health study shows that your belief that stress hurts you may be the culprit that makes you sick. Instead, if you see your natural stress response as helpful in attending to the issues that cause you stress, your blood vessels do not constrict. And seeking support from those around you about your stressful situations actually protects your cardiovascular system and strengthens your heart.

It works the other way too. A University of Buffalo, Department of Psychology 2013 study showed that people who spend time supporting and caring for others showed no increase in their risk of dying from stress. Dr. Kelly McGonigal, who made these announcements at a September, 4, 2013 TED Conference, adds that by going after what creates meaning in your life, and by trusting yourself to handle the stress that follows, allows you to keep that stress from killing you.

So managing your ATTITUDE toward your stress may end up being be your most effective tool to manage your stress... which leads us to Step 7.

CHAPTER 11. STEP 7—ATTITUDE

As Charles Swindoll put it, "We cannot change the inevitable. The only thing we can do is play on the one string we have, and that is our attitude. I am convinced that life is 10% what happens to me and 90% how I react to it."

This chapter is all about enjoying your ride on the Longevity Express, not just pointing toward your destination. No matter what, if you don't enjoy the journey on some level, you'll most likely fall off the train. Ultimately, it's up to you.

In the original draft of this book, called *SALADS*, I covered six steps, not seven. In fact, that's how I came up with the name. SALADS stood for Supplements, Activity (exercise), Lifestyle, Anti-Aging medicine and Stress management. Corny I know, but still semi-cool. At least I thought so. But there's an important seventh step that I am adding to the book. That step is Attitude. It messes up my original acronym, but it has a huge impact on your longevity.

I know a life extensionist who is facing more challenges now than most people face in a lifetime. Yet he remains upbeat and optimistic. I know a person who is not interested in extreme life extension who is crushed by a disruptive (but temporary) challenge, which has sunk him into a deep state of depression.

About 90% of the members of the life extension community I know would fit the first profile. They seem to function well in the face of adversity, bounce back from setbacks and are overall, healthier than average.

I find the majority of people with no interest in extreme life extension tend to react more negatively to challenges and also tend to be less healthy.

Then I came across an article by Paul J. Rosch, M.D. It illustrated how optimistic people live longer. Here are some excerpts:

> Numerous studies support the belief that people with an upbeat and positive perspective tend to be healthier and enjoy longer lives than those who are gloomy and cynical about the future. Always expecting the worst was linked to a 25% higher risk of dying before age sixty-five in a very long-term California study. In another report on senior citizens, researchers rated 1,000 Dutch men and women aged 65–85 with respect to their degree of optimism, health and longevity. Over the next ten years, participants classified as being very optimistic had 55% fewer deaths from all causes and 23% less heart-related deaths than highly pessimistic controls.

So Stay Happy and Save Your Life

> The article cites study after study proving optimism extends your life. For example, it goes on to say:
> Harvard researchers found cardioprotective effects when they followed 1,306 men who had been rated for optimism and pessimism in 1986. During the next ten years, men reporting high levels of optimism had almost half the risk of suffering any coronary complications compared to peers classified as being very pessimistic.
> Optimists and happy people may also be less likely to suffer a stroke according to a University of Texas study of 2,478 senior citizens. Researchers confirmed that increasing depression ratings were associated with a significantly higher incidence of stroke.
> Similar rewards were reported in a study of 600 people over age fifty in a small Ohio town in 1975. Researchers found that optimists who viewed aging as a positive experience lived about 7.5 years longer than participants with a much darker perspective.

One might argue that people in poorer health would be more apt to have negative responses and also be more likely to die over the next twenty-three years.

However, even when health, socioeconomic status, overall morale, loneliness, race, sex, and other possible confounding factors were taken into account, a positive view of aging was still highly correlated with significantly increased longevity. Indeed, this advantage was far greater than that afforded by lowering blood pressure or reducing cholesterol, each of which was found to lengthen life about four years.

In a Mayo Clinic study, optimists:

- had fewer limitations due to physical health.

- had less pain.

- felt more energetic most of the time.

- felt more peaceful and happy most of the time.

- had fewer problems with work or other daily activities as a result of their emotional state.

Over and over, I see evidence of how attitude contributes to health and longevity. If you look for the correlation, you'll find it, too. But more importantly, look within.

Dr. Arnold A. Hutschnecker, author of *The Will to Live* says: "Aging is mainly psychological, not biological. Everything in our society tells us that as we grow older, we will lose our mental powers, our health, our sexual capacities. We start believing it all, and because we believe it, it begins to come true. But it doesn't have to be this way. Seventy-five percent of so called aging results from a self-fulfilling prophecy."

The Placebo Effect

Thousands of reports demonstrate how positive attitudes helped patients rid themselves of all sorts of diseases, including cancer. And most of us are familiar with the "placebo effect." During double-blind studies, patients are often randomly selected to get a drug or a sugar pill for the term of the study. The purpose is to determine which group, if any, responds positively. If the patients getting the drug show improvement, then that could be strong evidence that the drug works.

However, the groups getting the placebo often improve as well. That's because they don't know they are getting a sugar pill. They may think, or hope, they are getting some new miracle drug that is going to cure them. So, many of them improve simply because of their attitude.

Science has proven you're wired for direct connections between your thoughts and emotions and your health. We were brought up with a healthcare system that focuses on drugs and the illusion of quick fixes, and one that mostly ignores the powerful mind-body link. Modern medicine tends to assume we feel a certain way because of our physical condition. It misses the fact that how we feel is actually the cause of our physical condition.

The placebo effect is actually a *perception* or a *belief* effect. The history of medicine is largely the history of the placebo effect. Arthritic knees are one example. In one study at the Houston Veterans Affairs Medical Center, Baylor College of Medicine, the placebo effect (fake surgery) improved patients just as much as the other two groups who received surgery. In more than half the clinical trials for the six leading antidepressants, the drugs did not outperform sugar pills. There are thousands of other examples.

When the mind, through positive suggestion improves health, it is referred to as this placebo effect. Conversely, when the same mind is engaged in negative suggestions that can damage health, the negative effects are referred to as the *nocebo* effect. Doctors' words and actions can trigger both. You can live or die because you believe you will live or die, and doctors can be responsible for their patients recovering or even their dying by the messages they communicate to them.

The messages you receive, the messages that reach your cells are the key. You are the gate keeper. To thrive, you need to actively seek a joyful, loving and fulfilling life that stimulates growth. Examine how your fears and the ensuing protection behaviors impact your life. Are any fears stunting your growth? Where did they come from? Are they necessary? Real? Are they contributing to a full life, or are they shortening it?

You can change long-standing limiting beliefs in a matter of minutes. Read *Biology of Belief* by Dr. Bruce Lipton to learn more about the cure-all we were born with but too often use in reverse.

An interesting UCLA study demonstrated that by consciously shifting from one emotional state to another, actors could stimulate or suppress their immune systems. Subsequent studies showed changes in hormone levels, blood sugar levels and wound healing abilities are all affected by emotional states. So when you simply decide to be happier and replace toxic negative thoughts with positive thoughts, you will improve your health.

Your thoughts and emotions hold this powerful influence over your physical health. In fact, the link between emotion and cancer is so strong that some psychological tests are better predictors of cancer than physical exams. And there's also a strong link between emotions and cancer survival.

Finally, it has been proven that the simple act of *deciding* to take action to improve your health leads to measurable physical improvement. This is another example of the placebo effect. Just the act of reading this book and deciding to incorporate some or all of the seven steps to your longevity will make you healthier. Then when you follow-through, you close the deal.

Dr. Pete Hilgartner

What is your first reaction to a crisis? Let's say you get diagnosed with a serious illness. First your heart skips a beat and then thunders like a jackhammer. Maybe you break out in a cold sweat. Then when reality sets in, do you retreat? Do you roll up in a fetal position, pull the covers over your head and hope your problems disappear? Do you tend to sleep more, head for the liquor cabinet or pray harder than you had in years?

How about when your life's savings get wiped out overnight due to mismanagement, theft, the economy or just hard luck?

Or what do you do when the economy slows down, and your customers' orders slow to a trickle, or you get laid off?

What about when all the real estate equity you built over the years vanishes overnight?

Time to retreat, right? Batten down the hatches. Cut expenses. Downsize. Deprive yourself until things get better. That's what most people do, and that's one reason the press tells you our economy sucks.

What if there was a better way to handle crises? Well there is. In fact there are two. The first is offered up by Dr. Pete Hilgartner. The second is by yours truly.

Dr. Pete is a fascinating guy and a successful student of life. He was very sickly as a child, way sicker than most people could tolerate. But his illnesses motivated him to set lofty goals. He decided to win an Olympic gold metal, to become an officer in the Marine Corps and to become a physician. He was well on his way to a shot at the gold when his ailing back tripped him up. So he joined the Marines and later became a successful physician. Action at work!

The Marines taught him one of life's great lessons. They taught him how to survive an ambush.

Capt. Pete survived six ambushes in fact. He realized he survived them the same way he survived his childhood injuries and the same way he's surviving today's economic climate. When you're ambushed, the Marines teach you to head for an escape route. But what if there is none? What do you do when the enemy closes off all escape? Then you make yourself as small a target as possible, right? Wrong!

If you want to escape, to survive, you do the counter-intuitive. You do the unexpected. You expand, take action… and attack. But don't just sort of expand. Expand with decisiveness, purpose, order and with a plan. Play offense instead of defense. Overcome your fear, and take the fight to the enemy. Dr. Pete and most of the company he commanded live today because of that one critical lesson.

Have you noticed that when people are filled with fear, they tend to withdraw? They stop communicating. If they do communicate, it's usually to complain about how bad things are. When you're down or sick, become a beacon of optimism. Take charge of your situation. Every cell in your body will react and rally you to your recovery.

Can you force yourself to expand, when every fiber of your existence wants to do what everyone else is doing: succumbing and contracting to fear? Yes, you can. And you will!

I have another way to not only survive, but to prosper as well. It's your surest path to sound health and longevity. In a word, it's "prevention." Expand now, and avoid your ambushes. That's what Part II of this book is all about. Head off disease and illness by taking precautionary measures now and forever.

It's a well-known fact that people will do everything in their power searching for cures but will ignore preventative measures. Terminal diseases and what is happening now are concretes. The threat of disease and the future are abstracts. So we live for the moment while internal time bombs tick away. Sooner or later, one catches up with you. And more often than not, it's too late. If you catch it early enough and/or expand and attack, you have a chance to beat it back. But not all of Capt. Pete's soldiers got out alive.

Will tomorrow's technologies obsolete death from aging and other diseases? I'm certain of it. Will we all live to see the day? Unfortunately, no. And most of those who miss the extreme longevity boat will miss it because of inattention to prevention. Some will make it because they will expand when their crisis catches up with them. With so much at stake, why gamble? Stare fear in the face. Play to win, not to not lose. Expand right now, before it's too late.

Sure, living in fear of being dead may be irrational, but living in fear of chronic pain, degeneration and suffering seems totally rational to me.

You'd be terrified if a random thug could credibly threaten you with half the physical harm that aging is capable of. That's when you need to expand. Fear is a great motivator, but unfortunately far from reliable in what it motivates people to do. The various shadings of fear are well characterized by a loss of analysis and control. So most people withdraw and lightheartedly walk towards degenerative aging and its suffering. The vast majority choose to do nothing to try to avoid that future.

Now getting back to reacting to a health crisis. In case you haven't figured it out so far, I have some terrible news for you.

You have a terminal disease that no one has ever survived. It affects all your organs and tissues. You were born with it, and you too will die from it—unless you improve your odds by expanding and by preventing. It's our old adversary, aging. Instead of complaining about it, or even joking about it, for the first time in history, you can actually do something about it. One contribution many of us can make is supporting the research that will conquer the effects of aging while you are still alive. The other is simply taking a proactive approach to your condition to keep yourself alive until emerging medical miracles will give you a new lease on life.

When you wait for an emergency, it's usually too late. We work on your behalf to keep you ahead of the game. Why would you gamble with your greatest asset... your life?

You Own You

I recently met a man named Joel, a vibrant, energetic and successful businessman. He is an example of a person who turned his health condition around overnight. Even fanatical I am impressed and humbled.

Until 2007, he was on a happy unconscious lifestyle path. He had no interest in changing, in spite the overweight guy in the mirror. He was happy enjoying steak dinners and good wines almost every night at upscale New York restaurants.

He then had the good fortune to be asked by his daughter, and encouraged by his son, to go to a Tony Robbins life mastery retreat in Fiji. There, Joel became painfully aware of his annual weight gain trend, not exercising and over indulging with wine and toxic food. He realized if he wanted a future, he had to change and not wait for a (possibly fatal) crisis.

He says change comes from within, and outside influences like the food industry and business networking were no longer going to dictate his health standards. Since he was used to leading his business career, he decided to take charge of and lead his wellness too. By the time he left the seminar, he made a choice to make health his priority.

Joel immediately became a raw vegan and stopped all soda, coffee, prescription drugs and alcohol. One result of many? His weight dropped from 230 to 180. He has stayed with his new habits except for moderating his fully raw vegan diet. He does lots of fresh juicing and exercises 3 to 5 times a week.

The most important elements Joel would like to share with you are that we all work hard to create the success we have at whatever level that may be. And we have families and others we love and who love us. Therefore, we must be conscious about the stress we allow in our lives, how we treat ourselves and others, and how we view life's circumstances.

We are NOT the conditioning of our parents, and we aren't even our genetics. We're the masters of our domain and environment, and we personally get to determine how we treat our bodies, minds and emotions. As we accept personal responsibility for those choices, we expand and grow in magnificent ways.

Joel goes on to say that love, laughter, health and gratitude get better and better. And his most important decisions were to make wellness and connection to God/source/life energy priorities, and to treasure each moment.

Joel did it, and so can you. You don't even have to turn your habits around on a dime like he did. The more the better, but ANY improvement can enhance you and avoid future disaster.

Then there's Stanley Bronstein, a successful attorney and CPA who has lived most of his life being massively obese. On February 1, 2009, all that changed. Upon waking, he turned to his wife and said enough was enough. He said he was going to stop tolerating nonsense in his life and the first person he was going to stop tolerating it from was himself.

Almost 5 years later, he's gone from a weight of 320 pounds to 190, all by eating better and walking. His blood pressure's gone from a systolic in the 180s down to 95/55. His life has changed drastically as a result. Based upon pure statistics, he's probably added at least 8 years to his life and has certainly improved his quality of life as well.

Like many people who have drastically changed their lives, he's become devoted to helping others do the same.

Stanley says that until we're mentally willing to do what it takes, for the rest of our lives, any changes we make (including weight loss) will probably be temporary at best.

Stanley actively blogs about changing your life and consults with any who want to change their lives. You can read about his activities and philosophy on his website at: www.SuperChangeYourLife. com.

Can Expectations Determine How Long We Live?

I believe lots of us actually die because of our expectations. We're conditioned to believe the average lifespan is around eighty years, so we wind down and die right on schedule. We usually get what we expect, not what we want. What if you expected to live to 100? Wouldn't you naturally gravitate toward the habits that will make that happen? Wouldn't your thoughts and emotions be more positive? How about longer than 100 years? Loads of research tells us we should stay robust for up to 100. But why don't we? Could it start with your attitude? Don't cop out by blaming it on your genes or on luck. Really, 65–75% of it is the choices you make. Your genes account for less than 35%.

This is backed up by hard science. Studies have shown that people who just think they are aging faster actually do age faster!

If you always think the glass is half full, you're on the right track. Mayo Clinic research shows that people with positive outlooks typically live 19% longer than people who see the glass as half empty. It's questionable if this can be attributed to optimists being more likely to seek medical help when they're ill, or if their immune systems strengthen as a result of their sunny outlook. The end result is, they live longer. Optimists are also less likely to suffer depression and helplessness than their pessimistic counterparts.

To support the hypothesis that their immune systems are actually strengthened, Dr. Bruce Lipton's experiments, and that of other leading-edge scientists, have examined in great detail the processes by which your cells receive information. The implications of this research radically change our understanding of life. It shows that genes and DNA do not control your biology. Instead,

DNA is controlled by signals from outside your cells, including the energetic messages emanating from your positive and negative thoughts.

You can actually modify your genes without changing their basic blueprint by modifying their environment through changes in your diet, emotions, toxins, stress, etc. And guess what? Those modifications can be passed on to your future generations.

This process is called epigenetics. Science Daily defines epigenetics as a rapidly growing research field that investigates alterations in gene expression caused by mechanisms other than changes in DNA sequence. These patterns of gene expression are governed by epigenetic "marks" that sit on top of our DNA that tell our genes to switch on or off. These epigenetic "marks" cause certain unfavorable genes, like genes for obesity to express too strongly.

If you've already passed these legacies on to your children, they can undo much of the damage you caused them by following good lifestyle habits and keeping them from passing your garbage on to your grandchildren.

Everything you eat, drink, breathe, think and expose yourself to affects your genes. Those foods, beverages, toxins and *thoughts* trigger your genes to act in certain ways, either good or bad.

Scientists have discovered it is easier to make epigenetic changes than to fix damaged genes. Your epigenome is easier to mess up—but it's also easier to fix. For instance, why does one identical twin develop cancer and the other remain healthy when they have identical DNA? Why does one twin become obese and another remain lean? You have more control over yourself than nature has dictated through your genetic makeup.

Understanding how your cells respond to your thoughts and perceptions illuminates your path to personal empowerment. This largely determines how you look and feel and how long you live. In fact, only about five percent of cancer and cardiovascular patients can attribute their disease to heredity.

In his best-selling book, *Biology of* Belief, Dr. Bruce H. Lipton describes how biology's central dogma, that your genes control your life, contains one fatal flaw—genes cannot turn themselves on or off.

When cells are ailing, look first to the cell's environment for the cause, not to the cell itself. In a healthy environment, cells thrive. They falter in sub-optimal environments. The flow of information in biology starts with an environmental signal. Then it goes to a regulatory protein which goes to your DNA, RNA, and the end result, a protein. And you regulate this with the world's best "cure all," your mind.

The seemingly separate subdivisions of the mind, the conscious and subconscious, are interdependent. The conscious mind is the creative one that can conjure up positive thoughts. In contrast, the subconscious mind is a repository of stimulus-response tapes derived from instincts and learned experiences. The actions of your subconscious mind are reflexive in nature and are not governed by reason or thinking. It is strictly habitual; it will play the same behavioral responses to life's signals over and over again. How many times have you found yourself going ballistic over something trivial like another driver cutting you off in traffic? That's an example of a simple stimulus-response of a behavior program stored in your subconscious.

Endowed with the ability to be self-reflective, the self-conscious mind is extremely powerful. It can observe any programmed behavior you are engaged in, evaluate your behavior, and consciously decide to change your program.

Programmed behavior can come from almost anywhere. Once you accept the perceptions of others as "truths," their perceptions become hardwired into your own brain. What if they are wrong? What if your teachers give you destructive programming? What if the news reports you get are slanted? Your subconscious works only in the "now." Programmed misperceptions in your subconscious mind are not monitored and will habitually engage you in destructive and limiting behaviors. You can actively choose how to respond to most environmental signals and to control your beliefs. You can even choose to not respond at all. Your conscious mind's capacity to override your subconscious mind's preprogrammed behaviors is the foundation of free will.

Dr. Lipton concludes that beliefs control biology.

He clearly describes the connection between your core thoughts, beliefs and attitudes and how your cells function as a result. Happy thoughts put your cells' functions in balance. Hateful, angry and resentful thoughts do the exact opposite. They suppress your immune system, alter your hormones, upset your digestive system, and diminish your brain function and respiration.

Dr. Lipton's profoundly hopeful synthesis of the latest and best research in cell biology and quantum physics is being hailed as a major breakthrough showing your body can be changed as you retrain your thinking.

Finally, an often repeated study showed that when a person's living cells from different organs are put in separate dishes, cells from one organ would respond when cells from a different organ in a different dish were stimulated. If the cells were from two different people, they would not get the reaction. This means the trillions of cells in your body are always in direct communication with one another, even if they are not in direct contact by chemical or neurological pathways.

Stub a toe, and all your cells react. Poison your body with cigarette smoke or toxic food, and you stimulate every cell. Subject yourself to uncontrolled stress, and you stress tens of trillions of cells. Now can you see why stress management and attitude are so critical to your health and longevity?

Now that you know your thoughts affect every single cell in your body, what are you going to do about it? Since you now realize positive, loving and grateful thoughts keep you healthy and make you live longer, while negative thoughts destroy you from the inside out, you have a big anti-aging advantage. What happens to you usually doesn't matter one bit. How you react means everything.

I don't care what your situation is. You have plenty to be grateful for. I know I do. When things go awry, it's natural to be consumed by them and to forget all the wonderful things you have going for you. I have lots of positive things and people in my life, and sometimes I slip and take them for granted.

I've been fortunate enough to have attracted better friends, partners and relationships than most could ever hope for. And except for my injury, I lucked out in the health department. Then there are the little things I also tend to take for granted. For example, I started the day with a nutritious, delicious breakfast and ended it with a fabulous dinner. I live in one of the best climates in the world. I have a warm comfortable bed. My shoes fit. I have shoes. I have feet. And I have a couple of pages of other things to be grateful for, and so do you. Just writing this makes me feel a lot better, because when you think a grateful thought, there's no room in your mind for anything else.

So happiness could be as simple as deciding what you want to dwell on. And happiness equates to wellness. And good health leads to longevity and to even more happiness. Sure, you have to face your problems. But when you do, think of solutions rather than dwelling on the negatives. You can never have true happiness without good health.

Still having a hard time being happy? Then try this. Smile. Yes, that's right. Just smile. When you do, it's almost impossible to be unhappy. Smiling actually sends positive chemical and neural signals to every cell in your body.

How Food Can Affect Your Attitude

It doesn't always take just a positive mental state to improve your attitude either. Your attitude can also be affected by what you eat. Good nutritious food can give you a strong attitude, which in turn can help heal you. Conversely, unhealthy food (what most people eat) can often affect your attitude in a negative way and contribute to your sickness. These attitudinal effects are in addition to the beneficial or detrimental effects the foods have on your body.

The same holds true for drugs, supplements and supplemental hormones.

Let me tell you two personal stories that illustrate how big an impact some of these can have on you.

I Didn't Care Anymore

Several years ago, I slid into a deep funk. It happened over a period of a week or so, and lingered for a couple of weeks before I discovered what caused it. During those weeks, I could barely get out of bed. All I wanted to do was sleep. I had no energy or motivation and got to the low point where I didn't care if I lived or died.

Now that was a major event in my life, since I am Mr. "do everything you can do to stay alive." The only time I experienced that kind of negativity was after a spinal cord injury paralyzed me. It took me a good while to turn my attitude around then. But in some ways, this was even worse. I had no idea what was happening to me and finally went to a lab to get a blood panel done. The results were startling. My liver enzymes were off the charts, and my hormones were way out of whack.

Since I supplement with fairly high doses of niacin, my liver enzymes gave me a clue. I had changed niacin brands a month or two earlier and dug out one of my new niacin bottles. What I discovered blew my mind.

The old niacin tablets were 100 mg. The new capsules were 1,000! Ten times the dosage—and I was taking several capsules 3 times a day. I didn't notice the increased dosage, because I dump my supplements out of the bottles into a convenient vitamin case. Then I stopped taking niacin altogether and within a few days, I was completely back to normal with my previously positive attitude intact. I'm back to my original dosage now but with it all bundled into one daily dose. I also found out that spreading niacin out during the day can be tough on your liver.

The World's Angriest Woman

I knew a woman who would wake up mad at the world and go to sleep madder yet. Almost everyone who crossed her path, even slightly out of line, would incur her wrath. You did not want to be near her. Any sane person would avoid her like the plague after one close encounter.

Then an interesting thing happened. She changed. Now she wakes up with a song in her heart and with nice words for all (well, almost all). She's happy, pleasant to be around and no longer a threat to fragile egos.

As it turns out, she was, shall we say, hormonally challenged. She too had some blood work done. And her results were startling as well. Her hormones were so far off balance that her physician tactfully told her she suffered from an extreme case of a common malady. But he tamed the beast with simple hormone replacement therapy.

These two examples show how reducing a supplement got my hormones, and my attitude, under control and how taking supplements (hormones) got my friend's hormones, and her attitude, under control.

These illustrations are also two good reasons to see an anti-aging physician who is qualified to check and monitor your hormone balances. It's not just for women. As men age, they typically suffer from abnormal hormone levels, too, which in turn affect attitudes, vitality and even body shape.

So your attitude, which could affect your longevity, can stem from what you put in your mouth and from out-of-balance hormones. There's more to attitude than just managing your thoughts. Stay positive, live long and prosper—and get regular checkups and blood panels.

Sense of Purpose

Having a strong sense of purpose goes a long way to improving your outlook on life and on your attitude. In fact, without a clear sense of purpose, extreme life extension may turn out to be an empty dream. Make a commitment to a life-long purpose. Be driven, even relentless in your determination to do or discover something. Your mission may be inspired by faith, conventional religion or personal convictions. It may be working on an important problem like, "Why do we get old and die?" or "How does the brain work?" or "What can I do to end starvation?" or simply "What can I do to help ensure the health, wellbeing, success and happiness of all my family members?" or any other worthy purpose.

Choose a mentor, a personal hero/heroine or someone to emulate. Find a mentor or mentors who live positive healthy lives. Pick their brains. When you think what a health-oriented person thinks, you become healthier. The fastest way to change any habit is to act as if it is already true.

Become a mentor. Pass your mentor's knowledge on to your students when they're ready, in order to create a multigenerational legacy. As Scaramouche once said, "I must now learn from the teacher of my teacher."

Another way to boost your sense of purpose and outlook is increasing your spirituality. Join a church and go to services at least on annual holidays. Other ways are: meditate regularly; look at the positive sides of life—stay optimistic and flexible; have a sense of humor about adversity; laugh and tell jokes; watch funny movies; develop a strong social network; go out socially once a week; find someone with whom to share your personal feelings and problems.

Sing songs, listen to music, play an instrument.

Stay informed without getting consumed by negative news: Watch TV news sparingly. Listen to the radio. Scan newspapers. Read magazines, journals and books and surf the Internet. Go to a local library. Go out to the movies at least once a month. Rent CDs, DVDs or download your entertainment. Go to the theater/ballet/opera/symphony/concert at least a few times a year. Keep mentally active: play chess, checkers, cards, video games or Scrabble. Go to school and take courses. Go to lectures. Go to museums.

Finally, do what you love, and love what you do.

"Good Ideas, I'll Start Tomorrow"

Do you find yourself waiting for the "perfect moment" to start? Maybe the time to start will be "tomorrow." Then ask yourself this question. Was there ever a time when you let an opportunity slip by when you could have taken action—but didn't? I know I have. And it hurts. Now remember a time when you went for it and succeeded. Exhilarating, wasn't it? So why don't we unleash empowering action more often? Why do we procrastinate and pretend there is plenty of time? Fittingly, in this case, procrastination will *cost* you time. It will cost you the extra years of youth that *Smart, Strong and Sexy at 100?* promises you. Your life. Your time. Your choice.

How many times have you started on a new diet or exercise program only to end up back to where you started, or worse? Was

motivation the missing element? The hardest part of any new program is the insidious mental resistance that sabotages us. Well, I've
got good news for you. Once you start Longevity Express' seven-
step program, you *will* want to continue, naturally and unforced.
You'll love the process as well as the results. It will be enjoyable
instead of work. It will become as much a part of you as getting
dressed in the morning, regardless of your age or fitness level.

Ride the Express to a destination where staying healthy, strong
and fit stops becoming "what you do" and turns into being "who
you are." See yourself congratulating yourself when you reach
this exhilarating point of freedom. See yourself as healthy, fit and
happy. Be patient.

Mastery takes time. You'll use regular motivation during the
journey, but you won't depend on it forever. The longer you ride
the Express, the easier and more enjoyable the ride becomes.
Soon, you will love the process and break free from the pro-aging
habits that used to ruin your life and pointed you to an early grave.

Vibrant, youthful life is simply a superior alternative. You'll get
to the point where not doing what you should be doing to maintain your vitality and longevity will be much more painful to you
than just doing it will be. You won't need to depend on willpower
and discipline except to create your original rituals. Then you'll
be on auto-pilot.

Think about it. Once you learn to read, would you ever revert
to illiteracy? Learning to read is transformative. You'll never go
back. It's the same with learning to control your wellness and longevity. Once you learn how and experience the wondrous benefits,
turning back will simply be unthinkable. You don't need more discipline. You need more rituals.

We don't like it when our actions conflict with our thoughts.
That makes us very uncomfortable and makes us prone to change
our actions. Think healthy—be healthy.

However, if you know you should book a seat on the Express
but it doesn't connect enough with you to start seriously, simply
don't do it. Just make sure you completely understand what you
are passing up. The Express could easily transport you from an
ugly premature death to an era where suffering and aging are left

far behind—to an era where you could enjoy open-ended youth, strength and vitality.

Here are a few mental tricks to help get you there:

- Remind yourself of your successes.

- Visualize your future.

- Think about what means most to you.

- Make your plans realistic.

- Think about things that energize you.

- Give yourself compliments.

- Expect the best.

- Realize change is possible.

- Imagine yourself aging more slowly—or even growing younger.

- Feel in control, trust yourself.

- Live consciously.

- Accept what comes your way and deal with it.

- Forgive yourself and others.

Illness and Disease

How about if you already have a health challenge? If you are faced with an illness or disease, here are some ways you can use the power of your brain to improve your chances of recovery:

- Don't think about the pain.

- Concentrate on getting better.

- Believe in your treatments.

- Imagine your strong immune system.

- Picture your body fighting off infections.

- Listen to your body.

- Find a positive and friendly doctor.

- Believe in miracles.

- Don't fear treatments.

- Relax.

- Start thinking of yourself as a healthy person.

- Don't milk injuries.

- Understand that sometimes it's all in the mind.

- Don't expect pain.

- Don't place blame for illness.

Imagination Always Trumps Willpower

Willpower is the conscious part of you that you put to work when you are determined to do something. The sheer force of will can move mountains, at least in the short run. But used alone, willpower almost always fails.

Imagination puts your unconscious mind to work to transform your thoughts into reality. Virtually every major value sprung into existence only after it was first imagined.

How often have you heard the link between willpower and staying on a diet or willpower and sticking to a training routine? Unless you first anchor the willingness to eat properly or to stick to regular exercise to imagination, you will most likely fail. That's why most people gain weight back as fast as they lose it and why so many health club memberships go unused.

Here's all you need to do to succeed from now on:

See yourself as you want to be. Imagine enjoying your ideal lean powerful body. See yourself as lovable, energetic, attractive and happy. Imagine being as fit as you want to be. Keep these images in your mind constantly. Visualize them just before you nod off to sleep and right after you wake up in the morning.

Monitor your thoughts. If you notice a negative or unhealthy thought, immediately replace it with a positive strong thought. Your mind will not be able to hold more than one thought at a time. When you think it does, it is actually jumping from one thought to another.

So put self-talk to work for you. You are constantly talking to yourself. Your subconscious remembers every word and eventually transforms those words into reality.

What do you want your reality to be? If you want to eat well and if you want to stick to regular exercise routines, see yourself doing so, and imagine your ideal results. Once you permanently establish these pictures in your mind, you naturally gravitate to the activities and habits that deliver you your rewards.

You will see it from the outside, only after you see it from the inside. No stress. No mess. No willpower needed. Until you replace your old negative images with your new positive images, you will continue finding reasons to abandon your diet and to skip workouts.

If you don't believe me, listen to Einstein who said "Imagination is more important than knowledge."

Are you ready to book your ticket on the Express? If so, you must take action *now*, because tomorrow never seems to come. Then what's the best way to stay in action? Diligently measuring and tracking your activities' progress. To successfully manage your aging, it's vital to keep a daily log.

TRANSFORMATION MEASUREMENTS

	Day 1	30 Days	60 Days	90 Days	120 Days
*Skin Elasticity					
*Reaction Time					
*Static Balance					
*Vital Lung Capacity					
*Memory/Cognition					
Weight					

Body Fat %					
Blood Pressure					
Resting Heart Rate					
Blood Glucose					
Hormones					
Homocystine					
Fibrinogen					
HDL/LDL Ratio					
C-Reactive Protein					

*See Introduction for at-home tests.

How do you keep yourself on track for 120 days… and beyond? In his book, *The 4 Hour Body*, Tim Ferris offers four principles of failure-proofing behavior.

1. **Make it conscious.** Use and follow the Transformation Measurements chart I give you here. And if you're trying to gain or lose weight or change your body shape, take unflattering before photos in a bathing suit or in your underwear. Then keep them visible as your constant reminder.

2. **Make it a game.** Set specific goals. Set your sites low to start, setting easy short-term goals. Make it a point to do something five times. Measurement equals motivation, so keep track, and gradually move on to more ambitious goals. And let yourself and your actions be observed by friends or family.

3. **Make it competitive with public recognition.** This way, you expose yourself to tangible risk of public failure. But keep it friendly, and compete with friends and family who share your common goal. Understand that a potential loss is a greater motivator than a potential reward. Instead of rewarding yourself with success (achieving your goals will

be your reward), set yourself up to lose something if you don't succeed.

4. **Make your initial goal small and temporary.** Don't try to bite off too much at first, and create momentum. Take the pressure off by doing something small. Get started on at least two changes. Then take baby steps by starting with one to two week goals. Finally, make your first five sessions as painless as possible.

Tim goes on to say "Track it, or you will fail." So there you have it. Once you start measuring your progress, it won't be long before you fall into new positive habit patterns. This wisdom goes way back to Aristotle, who said "We are what we do repeatedly."

That wraps up the Longevity Express 'seven steps. Climb aboard now, and you will overcome or mitigate much of the genetic bad hand you might have been dealt. We have learned we are not as governed by our genetic makeup as we once thought. As it turns out, your lifestyle determines much more of how you end up than your genes do.

It simply boils down to a matter of personal choice. Your future's biggest determining factors are the decisions you make now. Your choices make up who you are, how you end up, and in this case, how long you will live. You are not controlled by your genes, your environment or your associates. You are a product of the choices you make, plain and simple. So take charge of your life and your future now.

You'll Look and Feel Great—and for Longer, too.

The Express promotes optimal health and vitality through every level of life. There's no reason to "feel like sixty" when you can feel like thirty or forty. Then it won't be long before "100 is the new 50."

Eighty is already the new fifty. It really is for those who take care of themselves. Just follow these seven steps, and you'll see. The next step, "100 is the new 50," will soon follow. After that...?

Do you want to look great—or look great "for your age?" Do you want to feel great—or feel great "for your age?" There's a huge difference.

Now you might be thinking, this sounds like a lot of work. It might also seem like these habits will take time away from your work or family. The truth is exercise and stress reduction techniques, along with a sensible diet and supplements, will give you more energy and better sleep patterns. They make you more effective, more efficient and more productive in less time. The net result is, you should have as much time as you have now for your normal activities—but more weeks, months and years to do the other things that are important to you.

I think it was Einstein who first said it. "Insanity is doing the same thing over and over again and expecting different results."

People will do almost anything to stay in their comfort zones. But if you want to accomplish anything, get out of yours. It will take a little effort—but not as much as you might think.

Hell on Earth Would be Meeting the Person You Could Have Been

There is no waste and no regret greater than getting good advice and ignoring it. There's a price to pay for any improvement, advancement or achievement, and you won't see progress until you change something. In other words, there is no free lunch. But people hate effort and get stuck in mediocrity, obesity, lethargy and sickness.

You might not be ready for this message, and you might not be ready until disaster strikes. I hope not. The sad truth is people will typically go to the ends of the earth to cure something that goes wrong, but will spend little if any time, money and effort for prevention, even though preventative measures typically cost only 1/15 as much as cures. There are psychological reasons for this insanity— but no rational reasons. Therefore, my job is a tough sale. But it's a rational one—and a critical one. I could find lots of easier things to do with my life—but nothing more important. I'm totally convinced if you ride the Longevity Express, you'll extend the quantity and quality of your life—and possibly save it in the process!

This information definitely can and will avoid suffering and save lives. Will one be yours? If I can enhance or save your life, I've accomplished a big part of my mission.

Imagine it being ten years from now, and you ignored all the good advice in this book. Imagine lying in a hospital room, staring at the ceiling, connected to machines and with tubes sticking out of you. Think about how you would regret not having boarded the Express and taking that pleasant ride to a healthy future.

Now fast forward ten years from today, after you boarded the Express. See yourself, fit, lean and tan, jogging on a tropical beach.

Ninety-five percent of people simply do not think of the future very much. Far off events such as cancer, heart disease, death… and extreme longevity seem abstract to most, so they do little to prevent or encourage them today. They're usually more concerned with scratching itches than planning for tomorrow. So they go through life in a reactive mode rather than in a proactive planning mode. The soothing effects of a cigarette, the extra helping and rich dessert at dinner and the temptation to just kick back are too gratifying to resist. That's why so many people are sick, fat, out of shape and broke.

Then, all too often, and often too late, they get a wake up call. Their partner loses respect for them and leaves, or they have (and survive) a heart attack or stroke, get diagnosed with cancer or another killer disease, or a close family member or friend suddenly dies. Then they finally turn to a healthy lifestyle, hoping they can make up for a lifetime of destructive habits.

Do you want to become the driver on the road to a healthy, vibrant life instead of a passenger on the road to an abbreviated future? I think we both know the answer to that question.

How Hard Can This Be?

Let's take a look at the concepts of prevention and effort, and see if we really do take the easy way out when we get lazy.

Did you know real regrets only come when you don't do your best? Think about it. Half-hearted efforts give you half-hearted results. Ironically, life is actually easy when you live it the hard way—and hard if you try to live it the easy way. In other words, the rewards so far outnumber the effort that you end up cheating and hurting yourself if you try to take the easy path. Or as Muhammad Ali put it, "Suffer now and live the rest of your life like a champion."

So if you start getting negative or lazy, catch yourself and throw up a mental picture that motivates you to healthy habits that lead you to a long youthful life. Once you look at it this way, you will have an easier time staying on track.

Backing off from time-to-time is human nature. Accept it. You're not alone. When you are tempted to skip a workout or eat junk food, understand this happens to almost everyone. But remember, everyone who ever stopped exercising started by "missing once" and broke the habit of training. When you're tempted, here's what to do: Understand that the last workout you did may be the last one you will ever do. Imagine not ever eating well or being healthy again, because when you miss a step, that makes it easier to miss the next step. Pretty soon, you're fat, out of shape and self-destructing.

Long-term vitality and longevity is not a physical issue, it's a mental one. Missing any one step will not hurt you physically. It will however, chip away at you mentally. So recognize the potential consequences, and visualize positive images of your future self.

Everything you do or think sends a signal to your brain. Your brain then responds by releasing hormones and biochemicals that control your growth, repair, sex drive, energy and immune function. When you exercise regularly, supplement sensibly, eat well and meditate, positive signals go to your brain. Then your brain sends back positive signals to every one of the trillions of cells in your body.

Depending on your habits, you either grow younger biologically, age slower or age faster. Your brain doesn't watch a calendar. It judges your age on the signals you send to it.

Let's say you smoke like a chimney, lie around swilling beer and shoveling down potato chips and Twinkies. What kind of signals do you think you are sending to your brain? Those automatically trigger signals that shut down the processes of growth and life. That's because your brain gets messages that you are on the decline. Nature hard-wired you to age and die when it gets that input.

Let's say you do some things right though. You might exercise, but you still don't see any gains. If so, your diet or stress could be sending conflicting signals to your brain that cancel out most of your hard work. The name of the game is balance. When you balance all seven steps, you'll marvel at how the synergy among them propels you to levels of fitness, energy and youth that you have not experienced for years.

If your present habits are unhealthy and you continue them, what will your state of health be in ten years? Or in twenty? Will you be blind from not understanding how bad sugar is for you? Will you be unable to walk and talk because of the stroke you could have avoided by simply having your doctor monitor your fibrinogen level? Will you not know your own name or the faces of your closest family members because you ignored advice about eating healthy fats? How about the major heart attack or cancer you could have dodged by simply taking daily aspirin under a knowledgeable doctor's supervision? Cardiovascular disease is the leading cause of death in the US and one of the easiest to avoid. Will you even be alive in ten or twenty years? I hope so— and way beyond that.

I don't mean to be an alarmist. But several of my friends have died already. In almost every single case, they had habits that typically lead to the diseases that killed them.

Three days ago, one ex-smoker boyhood friend died a horribly uncomfortable death. Some others are suffering miserably from many of the conditions and diseases I described to you. Again, most, if not all could have avoided these conditions by following the seven simple steps in this book. You can master them quickly by combining some simple basic information with a dose of common sense and a simple desire to look and feel great.

Napoleon Hill, in *Think and Grow Rich*, identified sixteen traits that all successful people share. The top five apply to health success as well as business and personal success. Let's look at these five for a moment.

1. **Burning Desire.** Do you have a vivid vision of your desired future health?

2. **Superior Knowledge.** This is what you're getting here. You don't have to master any of this information. You just need instant access to it. And you can get that by keeping the Express as a reference manual, or by visiting www.MaxLife.org.

3. **Discipline.** Now you know exactly where to start and what to do.

4. **Decisiveness.** Napoleon Hill says to gather data, analyze information, make decisions on the spot, and stick to those decisions. Make an informed decision now to enhance your health and wellbeing. Why would anyone want to sacrifice long-term satisfaction for short-term gratification? You're in charge of your outcome. No one else is.

5. **All successful people surround themselves with a master-mind team or support group.** Share this information with your family and friends. Or, if you need support, we can give it to you. You don't need to know what the team members know. You only need access to an informed group such as Maximum Life Foundation.

So here's what you'll do. Ride the Longevity Express for three months. Fall off the wagon one or two days a week if you want. Start with a complete check-up including a blood panel with a good anti-aging doctor. Track your activities and your progress. Get tested again every month for the first three months. If you're a member of Life Extension Foundation, they offer professional inexpensive blood tests from virtually anywhere in the U.S. Visit www.lef.org/maxlife.

If you don't see and feel an amazing difference after three months, then go back to your old habits. But I know you'll continue—and tack on those extra 5–20 energetic years I promised you.

Before you go to sleep later tonight, think about how nice it will be when you regain your youth and vitality. The next time you get ready to pop a crispy French fry into your mouth, or whenever you crack the top of a sugar-laden soft drink, you'll realize this might be the one that pushes you over the edge to a heart attack or diabetes.

The more you think about French fries, cigarettes or soft drinks, the more you're going to want to eat a fresh salad or take a nice invigorating walk in the sun.

The more you put off exercise, the worse you feel. Soon you'll be enjoying the health that you now want. You're getting healthier, healthier and healthier.

How Much Action do You Need to Take?

The best healthy diet or routine is the one you stick to. Instead of shooting for perfection, shoot for improvement. Any improvement in your wellness and longevity is better than none.

Training twice a week and sticking to it is infinitely better than shooting for training six days a week and quitting. Ten minutes of exercise every day beats scheduling an hour a day and giving up.

If eating healthy seven days a week is unachievable for you, then do it three or four days a week and pig out the other days. If you can't bring yourself to eating well every meal, then do it every other meal, or all but one meal. Shoot for small continual improvements. Once you develop optimal habits part of the time, when you do the opposite, you will tend to gradually eliminate or cut back on the unhealthy meals and habits.

Either way, something is better than nothing, so don't get discouraged if you can't meet someone else's standards.

Refuse to Be Cheated by Death

How many times have you heard the expression "cheating death?" Hundreds? Thousands?

Every time you utter this expression, or even listen to it with acceptance, you disempower yourself. You give in to the "inevitable" and hope to cheat death temporarily by buying a little more time.

How about adopting the opposite mindset? Why not consider *yourself*, rather than death, being the unbeatable foe, and consider anything short of open-ended growth and vitality as being person-ally cheated?

Imagine entering a sporting event, a business transaction or a debate with the attitude that you hope to score a few points but are resigned to losing to a superior opponent. Why even try? If you're not trying to win, if you believe the best you can do is pick up a little concession here or there and are resigned to losing, what's the point?

However, I don't believe that's the way you live your life. By EXPECTING positive outcomes, you automatically adopt one of the more empowering tools available. The opposite is true as well.

Most of us expect to die from aging unless something else kills us first. What kind of attitude is that if you have an interest in con-tinual improvement? Positive expectations can move mountains. Negative expectations will help ensure you are buried beneath them.

Imagine betting your life on age-reversing research when the researchers are "sort of" "kind of" interested in slowing aging a little. Or how about the researcher who absolutely refuses to be cheated by death, whose unwavering mission in life is to crack the aging code and to deliver rejuvenating technologies to you in your lifetime? Which would you bet on?

How about the control you have over your own destiny? Do you agree it's possible to restore your youth in your lifetime? If so, are you doing everything in your power to keep yourself alive and sound long enough to take advantage? If not, reread the arguments in favor of radical life extension in Part I of this book. Before you can refuse to be cheated, you need to understand we are engaged in a winnable contest.

Seeing yourself age reinforces your resignation to aging and death. That's one reason why adopting the seven steps in this book is doubly important. You will *look* younger. See yourself differently too.

If that means you want to color your hair, get transplants, wear fashionable clothes and get cosmetic surgery... go for it. They won't make you stop aging, but they can slow down your resigna-tion to physical aging by tricking your psychological aging until the time when we can do away with aging altogether.

It's Not Your Fault

Now that you've seen the possibilities for longevity, health and happiness, are you unhappy with where you are now in relation to where you want your fitness level, appearance and health condition to be? Don't be. It's not necessarily your fault.

We weren't born smart, and most of the messages we're bombarded with come from providers of profitable but unhealthy products. Also, our teachers and physicians are usually uninformed as to what is and isn't good for you. That's also true of our governments. So the bottom line is, you didn't necessarily know. Life is a learning process, and we often get into trouble or in bad shape because of what we do not know.

But now that you do know what to do to recapture and preserve your health, vigor and looks, you can improve—starting now. Start with what you are learning here, and continue to educate yourself to make lasting changes.

If you're interested in keeping up-to-date with the most current longevity info that will give you more of what life offers, visit www.MaxLifeSolution.com and www.MaxLife.org/sssbook.

One Closing Thought

Look, the Longevity Express philosophy boils down to this:

For the first time in history, we have a shot at the brass ring. We have a chance to be part of the first generation to achieve open-ended growth—or to be a part of the last generation to die from aging. Your actions, starting today, may be the determining factor. Open-ended youth is right around the corner, so ask yourself this question:

How badly do you want it?

Only your actions answer that question. *Everything* is at stake. And the next section shows you how to empower yourself.

To maximize your chances for optimal health and longevity, take action now! Climb aboard the Longevity Express today.

Tomorrow never comes.

PART III

You Have More Power Than You Think

Whether you are charging ahead in life, standing still or falling behind, you are still ultimately falling behind biologically. Your habits just determine how quickly or slowly. In other words, there is no way you will live to even 110 without being seriously decrepit and without looking like crap. Only new discoveries can prevent or reverse that.

But you do have power over your destiny.

If your dream is renewed youth and vitality and a greatly extended upgraded lifespan, then you can make it happen. Are you taking charge of your health to increase your odds of staying alive and robust until future technologies will extend your active lifespan even more? Do you contribute to the research, either financially or intellectually? Do you donate any of your time and talents to Maximum Life Foundation or to another anti-aging group? In other words, are you moving forward boldly in life to help ensure your longevity?

Now that you have seen how and why open-ended growth is possible in our lifetimes and what you can do to boost your odds to benefit, let's talk a little about how much a project like this might cost.

First, some knowledgeable people think it will never be done in our lifetimes. Nearly every great advance was met with skepticism and derision. But breakthroughs are accelerating.

For those who do believe it is possible, projected timelines extend from something less than MaxLife's plan to as long as a hundred years. And some project the cost will be well over $1 trillion. How about you? What are your opinions? Can it be done? How long will it take? How much will it cost?

We have spent years pondering those questions and running calculation after calculation. After consulting with experts from all the disciplines we discussed in this book, after reviewing business plans and budgets and research plans and budgets, after factoring in the Law of Accelerating Returns and its Deflationary Factor, and after lots of educated guesswork boosted by optimism and tempered by the harsh reality of knowing projects usually cost more and take longer than we anticipate, here are our conclusions:

1. This is not a trillion dollar plus project. In fact, it's not even a $100 billion project, even though that would be one of the most incredible bargains of all time. (We spend that much on health care in the United States *every sixteen days*.) We came to the astonishing conclusion that we could accomplish enough to cure aging for the ridiculously low sum of $1.9 to under $5 billion, plus $900 million more for SENS (as described in Chapter Four). Total as little as $2.8 billion.

2. We can do this over a twenty-year span, starting from the time the first part of the funding is in place.

3. About $150 million a year may be all that is standing in the way of youthful open-ended lifespans.

4. This assumes no reinvested profits will be generated from any of the companies and technologies that would receive funding. If some of these were moderately successful, profits could be reinvested, which would reduce the overall cash outlay.

Another reason we should be able to control aging on a relatively tiny budget is, given unlimited time and money, people tend to approach problems the same old conventional way. However, limiting money and setting deadlines creates an urgent innovative environment where people think outside the box, try new approaches and tend to accomplish "the impossible" in record time. We have seen evidence of this among those who crafted our Scientific Roadmap to reverse aging.

In case it does cost a lot more, our budget will certainly result in proofs of concept so powerful that thousands, if not millions of investors will quickly grasp the profit and life extending implications. That will result in enough private sector investments to finish the job.

Ten thousand health-conscious individuals, just like you, could fund MaxLife's project for $1,200/month each. A handful of the ultra-wealthy could underwrite the whole project. And sophisticated private investors will have lots of choice opportunities to earn sizeable returns while contributing to their health and longevity. Meanwhile, MaxLife continues to identify many of these opportunities.

Better yet, we could lay the foundation for age reversal for about $60 million over three years and get a head start by launching some potentially explosive companies in one year for about $20 million.

If it costs so little, and even if it does cost over a trillion dollars, wouldn't this be something big business or governments would fund?

Unfortunately, "no," at least not now.

Historically, financial support for aging research and efforts to extend the healthy lifespan have been spotty. Venture capital firms typically aim for profitable exits from their investments within two to four years. The research and product development we support typically take longer to mature. Governments aren't providing much funding.

Pharmaceutical and biotech companies' support of basic aging research is hindered due to the fact that there are no generally accepted biomarkers for human aging that would allow the FDA to approve a drug designed to slow the aging process. These companies are forced to develop drugs for specific diseases. And the FDA doesn't recognize aging as a disease.

For example, *The New York Times* looks at Sirtris Pharmaceuticals: "The hope is that activating sirtuins in people would, like a calorically restricted diet in mice, avert degenerative diseases of aging like diabetes, heart disease, cancer and Alzheimer's."

Dr. Christoph Westphal, the former chief executive of Sirtris, said of the potential of the resveratrol-based drugs they developed, "I think that if we are right, this could extend lifespan by 5 or 10%." He added his goal was to develop drugs against specific diseases, with the extension of life being "almost a side effect of our medicine."

There is no FDA category for longevity drugs, so if the company is to submit a drug for approval, it needs to be for a specific disease. However, longevity is what has motivated the researchers and what makes the drugs potentially so appealing.

There you have the most serious problem facing longevity science today. The FDA does not allow its direct application. Until this policy changes, no serious investment will be made in the U.S. to bring longevity science to the clinic. This is a tragedy of astronomical proportions, and is beyond belief.

Congress did supplement scarce aging research dollars by establishing the National Institute on Aging in 1974, but that money has primarily gone to disease-specific research, such as Alzheimer's disease, or towards the behavioral aspects of aging.

So billions of dollars continue being squandered developing band-aid approaches to degenerative diseases instead of seeking to intervene directly in the underlying cause of these diseases, the aging process itself.

Consider This

What if all the funding for Alzheimer's, cardio-vascular disease, cancer and all the other aging-related diseases were halted and redirected toward life extension research?

Logically, healthy life extension is where it should go. Solve aging, and we avoid these other diseases. They mostly become non-issues.

Obviously, we won't do that. But what if we took a small fraction of those budgets and invested them in focused life extension research? Why aren't we doing that? If you look at it logically, not doing so is pure insanity. More pragmatically, the decision makers are simply not well enough informed. And there's a tremendous amount of inertia in the status quo. Ultimately, it's up to us to inform the public and to raise as much funding as we can, until we demonstrate a dramatic life extending or age reversal capability in lab animals. Then the investing world will get it, in spite of lack of government support.

In fact, if governments would just get out of the way, that could pave the fastest path to curing aging. For example, by comparing progress in medicine over the past thirty years with progress in computing and software, we can see a fraction of what might have been achieved by stripping away regulation, guilds, and central planning. Consider how primitive computers and their role in everyday life would look like if the computer industry had been regulated like medicine is today.

Introducing a new machine or new software package would have meant spending years and $100 million to pass a bureaucratic one-size-fits-all process. And radical new designs would have required a decade of expensive lobbying to be added to the list of what's permitted. A hundred thousand lives are lost every day to degenerative aging. But curative therapies will emerge at a snail's pace compared to how they would in a more open society than the one we have in the U.S.

How about all the other private money today? Where is it all going? Unfortunately, many popular investments may be ruining your health and shortening your life instead of extending it. And you may be unknowingly contributing to it. If you are invested in mutual funds, retirement funds or hedge funds, the chances are, you are invested in what I sometimes call "pro-death industries." They include fast foods, processed foods, alcoholic and soft drinks, and tobacco.

These industries make money—lots of it. That's why savvy money managers invest in them. But they kill in two insidious ways. First, the products can shorten your life. Second, they divert sorely needed funds required to develop life extending products, technologies and services.

Other industries are more benign. For example, ten years ago, hair dye was a $7 billion worldwide industry. A large fraction involves coloring gray hair. So it's not a stretch to suggest that the world's aging population have a great enough interest in hair dye to fund age-reversal research several times over.

This sort of comparison illustrates just how small research and development expenditures in medicine are in comparison to almost any form of day-to-day commerce. It's a mystery as to why people are so relentlessly irrational when it comes to directing resources towards actual improvements in health and longevity versus papering over the cracks with hair dye.

Is it the case that people decide between funding research and hiding the gray, and choose to hide the gray? Or is it that funding meaningful research doesn't really even enter that choice matrix? To reframe these questions, is the solution to funding the best and most promising longevity science more a matter of persuasion or more a matter of education?

Then, those with disposable income and assets donate to all kinds of charities, yet they overlook research that could help them live in a youthful state of health for a very long time. Again, a question of persuasion or education... or maybe both?

Assuming you understand the possibilities and the economics, doesn't it make sense to commit only a portion of your wealth to technologies that could cure diseases, promote wellness and extend your healthy life? Oh, did I mention that over a hundred times more money is spent on R&D for curing baldness than for curing aging?

The Most Important Person in the World... or... "If he's so smart, how come he's dead?" —Homer Simpson

You know how to boil a frog alive, right?

(Not that we want to...)

The secret is to gradually turn up the heat. If you make it real hot, real fast, the frog will jump out of the pot. But if you turn up the heat slowly, before the frog realizes it, it will be too late, and the frog slowly dies. As aging humans, we are all slowly (and some not so slowly) being boiled alive by the ravages of time.

What if we had a major sudden breakthrough in a technology that could make possible the complete rejuvenation of a human being, turning back the clock to optimum health and youth? Allowing for MORE time with family and friends and MORE time to achieve all of the goals one dreams of?

Making super sexuality a forever thing, not just a highly-charged stage of adolescent life? Going and doing and moving like a well-oiled machine once again? Don't you think aging billionaires, and anyone who could afford it, would make mad dashes to their checkbooks to complete the research before it's too late for them?

We don't have that breakthrough... yet! But it's on the horizon—just beyond our reach.

Our scientists say they KNOW how to do it, and in our lifetime. But that's contingent on funding.

Meanwhile, the world's 1,426 billionaires (total net worth over $5.4 trillion), like that ill-fated frog in the story above, are slowly being boiled alive. (In fact, Steve Forbes estimates there are actually about 3,000 billionaires.)

At some point it will become clear that aging to death while surrounded by wealth is insanity in an age where a fraction of those resources could be used to develop age-reversing medicine. But so far, this isn't obvious enough to those who can make a difference.

When it comes to access to medical technology, the world is remarkably flat. The wealthy have no more ability to buy a way out of aging presently than does anyone else. What they do have is a far greater ability to create a near future where rejuvenation technologies exist and are just as widely available as any present day clinical procedure.

Why, then, aren't they, or at least several of them, stepping up to the plate and getting out of the slowly heating "pot" that will put an end to all that they now enjoy and have worked so successfully to achieve?

After all, at least 248 of them have $5 billion or more, and we estimate we might solve aging for less than $5 billion total spread over the next twenty years. To put it in perspective, we spend more than that in the U.S. every day on a broken healthcare system.

For one thing, a proposal to fund the necessary research is out of the scope of their business or their favorite charity(s). After all, most high achievers at that level have diverse 1) business interests, 2) charitable activities and 3) investment portfolios.

But having what we're proposing as a focus makes little sense according to their traditional guidelines. The ONE SINGLE activity that could extend all three, supporting life extending research, better enables every other personal or business pursuit.

Let's analyze these three:

1. Business Interests – Anti-aging is an emerging trillion dollar industry. Entrepreneurs will build enormous companies, especially those who commercialize technologies that
   would dramatically extend the youthful portions of our
   lives, let alone reverse aging.

2. Charitable Activities – We lose 100,000 people to aging
   every single day. Then factor in the suffering. And how
   about the trillions of dollars of related medical costs? Then
   there are the social costs of continually losing our most productive and valuable minds. Learn how to control aging
   and we have pretty much solved heart disease, stroke, cancer, arthritis, etc.

   They're all important diseases to solve in themselves, but
   solve one, and another will probably get you. If you consider aging as a cause, and it is, then the others could be
   considered as symptoms. In other words, what could be a
   more impactful charitable contribution?

3. Investment Portfolios – Nearly every billionaire is invested
   directly or indirectly in some or all of the "pro-death" industries which I describe above. Another common thread is
   that they have virtually zero dollars invested in companies
   or technologies which will keep them from being slowly
   boiled to death. Isn't this seriously out of balance?

Youth is the Ultimate Wealth… and You're Poorer Today

We believe that once people know about emerging technologies that could dramatically extend the youthful portions of their
lives and their families' lives they will change the mix of their three
major financial activities. No one wants to suffer and die and to
see their families die when they have the power to avoid or at least
delay that. And that is the proposition we are engaged in.

Even if any thought there was just an outside chance for open-
ended youthfulness, they would probably be very interested in giving it a shot. And the worst thing that would happen to them is
there would be slightly less money for their heirs.

Some billionaires actually get it and in fact have offered some funding. But none has made a major commitment as far as I know. And that's tragic—for them and for you.

One of the reasons most billionaires amassed their fortunes is they have the gift of focus, of paying little attention to anything beyond their specialties. But this is one of those rare eras when so much hinges on paying just some attention to another field. The future of biotechnology has the potential to reshape and greatly extend all of our lives. Remaining ignorant or on the sidelines only adds to the chance that the necessary advances will arrive too late for them.

This isn't about any single person taking a plunge. On the other hand, someone who was able to single-handedly fund all the research, and completely change the world as we know it, would probably be recognized as "the most important person or company in the world." Certainly preserving 37 million lives a year would be worthy of that title.

More realistically however, the investments and donations will be spread among many. But those who step up to the plate now will be the ones who make the most impact. Every day's delay could ultimately cost up to 100,000 lives… they included.

The bottom line is… it completely baffles me why the world stresses and becomes obsessed over their businesses while they ignore extreme life extension endeavors. Building empires, investing, new innovations, competition, distribution, regulatory nightmares, administration, human resources and other activities consume business and financial leaders.

Then around eightyish, they die. How have their activities contributed to their wellness and longevity, or anyone else's for that matter? Except for the prospect of leaving something behind, what did it ultimately matter to them?

Please understand, I support and admire enterprise, contributions to society, a purpose of life and the commercial intricacies that enabled complex societies to develop and flourish. In fact, without them, we would not have reached this point… where controlling aging is finally possible.

Suddenly, the whole world is different. Transitory pursuits will still play key roles in our economies. But transitory they are, and transitory we are as long as we focus on traditional financial and business pursuits to the exclusion of life extension.

So let's not die rich because of inertia. Instead of planning on leaving a legacy, those with the financial means can now plan on LIVING their legacy if they so choose.

One such person may have made that choice in the fall of last year and another prior to that.

The first was Peter Thiel, cofounder of PayPal. He made a modest commitment and openly expresses his interest in seeing aging defeated. Let's hope this exceptional businessman's enthusiasm grows and he becomes a major player.

Next was was Larry Page when Google invested in a new company called Calico in September, 2013. Mr. Page implied that dramatically extending human life is one of Calico's main goals. The company has yet to release many details though.

Finally, on March 4, 2014, Dr. J. Craig Venter announced founding Human Longevity, Inc. (HLI). He is the most recent in a short list of famous entrepreneurs to tackle aging and aging related diseases. Dr. Venter is best known for being one of the first two to sequence the human genome and more recently, for creating the first cell with a synthetic genome. HLI was funded with $70 million in private capital, mostly from individual investors.

Google/Calico is of course the 800 pound gorilla. I'd feel better about their potential impact if their management wasn't so mainstream and institutional. They're competent business managers, but it would have been so much more encouraging to have seen some key managers with successful entrepreneurial track records and aggressive histories of passionate contributions to longevity research

As of this writing, it appears that Calico will primarily function as an R&D group, exploring the latest in longevity science. In the best case, they will apply laser-like focus on developing and bringing the key technologies to the clinics. In the worst case, they could set research back. Billions of lives are at stake.

When Google entered the picture, we heard some potential investors may have gotten scared off. They thought: "Well, why should we chip in when such big money started to work on this problem?"

But no company in the world can go in all of the directions that may lead to regulating biological clocks. Solving aging is incredibly complicated. It is unlikely one good idea or one company will do the trick.

And it's beginning to look like the world's billionaires may not need a driving quest for longevity in order to support the research either. More than any *decade* prior, this past year's involvement of Larry Page and Craig Venter helped open the eyes of the world to the potential enormous *profitabilability* of investing in this exploding sector.

This is the time to bear down, not to slack off. So let's hope Google's entry sets an example and encourages the rest of the world to follow their bold lead. One investor more or less, one research group joining or leaving, could swing the future timeline a decade or so in either direction.

What We are Doing to Reverse Your Biological Age

Bill Faloon, co-founder of Life Extension Foundation, and I independently thought of how to raise targeted funds for research. He brought up a concept while meeting with thought leaders at a medical conference in December 2008. Everyone acknowledged that potential advances might enable us to *reverse* the aging process we are all suffering. I attended the conference via telephone.

The problem was that no coordinated plan existed among the various scientific disciplines to collectively harness this technology into a near-term reality. He proposed we emulate what the United States did during World War II to rapidly develop the atomic bomb.

Coincidentally, I came up with the same proposal in June, 2000 at MaxLife's first international research conference in Manhattan Beach, California. We reasoned that if we instill a sense of confidence and urgency, we can collectively implement a "Manhattan Project" aimed at finding ways to reverse the festering aging process. Our project was aptly named the "Manhattan Beach Project."

Greta Blackburn and I followed up on Bill's suggestion and put together a "Longevity Summit" that consisted of some of the world's top anti-aging researchers. This conference titled "The Manhattan Beach Project – Longevity Summit" was held November 13–15, 2009, again in Manhattan Beach. The expenses were high because we had to fly gerontology experts in from around the world and cover hotel fees and video recording. Life Extension Foundation funded the entire cost, which amounted to around $60,000.

The first two days of this summit featured presentations by researchers who revealed their scientific roadmap for initiating and achieving *age reversal*. Most of these scientists had been quietly developing their technologies since our first conference. The last day was a roundtable discussion among the wealthy attendees, the scientists, and some very creative minds. The purpose of this brainstorm session was to develop plans to fund these anti-aging research initiatives that our lives so heavily depend on. The following consensus was reached:

1. In order to provide sufficient near-term funding to the most promising anti-aging research projects, about $100 million will need to be raised beyond what is already being spent by Life Extension Foundation and a few wealthy individuals who are currently giving money to gerontologists.

2. There are enough interested individuals today who are cumulatively able to provide this level of funding with moderate personal investments.

3. A company should be formed to not only raise and allocate these funds, but to also raise public awareness that a credible effort is being made to gain control over human aging.

A New "Age Reversal" Initiative

The first step in implementing the Manhattan Beach Project was to assemble a knowledgeable and experienced Board of Directors to assure that the new company would be competently managed.

The next challenge was lining up the seed financing to get this company off the ground. Initially, $2 million was raised from three investors, including Life Extension Foundation which provided $500,000.

We are now establishing a venture capital fund in addition to the company. The fund will accept investments from wealthy individuals and institutions to invest in the technologies such as those described in Chapter Four. The company will bring some of those technologies as well as current products and technologies to market. For information on either or both, please send an email to invest@MaxLife.org.

The primary motivation for people to be involved with this fund and company is, the research they support could lead to breakthroughs in controlling human aging. In turn, that could let them live much longer as well as better. The difference between this fund and company and others is the expectations of the investors. While we expect developing patented anti-aging therapies could yield considerable profits, that was not the main reason we thought individuals might participate.

Developing validated methods that would enable humans to grow biologically younger is far more valuable than all the money in the world.

The fund is set up to assist, both financially and technologically, companies whose research may lead to controlling human aging.

Not all of these age-reversal initiatives will pan out. But if just one led to the development of a validated method to *reverse* the course of aging, then every participant (and mankind itself) would benefit.

Age-Reversal Was Not Thought Possible

When Life Extension and MaxLife were founded, most people did not believe reversing human aging could ever happen. Now we know by showing that at least at the cellular level, it's possible to re-program genes to prompt human cells to go back in time. This discovery was announced in the June 2010 issue of *Life Extension Magazine*. Since then, progress has been snowballing.

When you look at the rapid technology advances we enjoy today, the probability of conquering aging can be easily analogized. Just think of the progress that has been made in other fields:

- From counting on fingers to supercomputers
- Riding on horse and buggies to flying on jet planes
- Waiting for the pony express to instant email and text messages
- Stage plays to satellite TV

One reason we are confident age-reversal is possible in our lifetime is the Law of Accelerating Returns described in Chapter Two. As scientists reach higher technological milestones, the accumulated knowledge base can be used to rapidly move up the scientific ladder.

At the Manhattan Beach Project – Longevity Summit, a number of scenarios for slowing or reversing aging were presented by eminent scientific authorities. The consensus among the participants was that it may be possible to cure aging in our lifetime. This prediction was made before a landmark aging reversal study was published in *Nature* just one year later (in November 2010).

We reasoned that if we could move up the next big anti-aging breakthrough by even a few years, this will mean the difference between life and death to many of those reading this book. That is why we tackle this mission with such a sense of urgency.

Where We Stand Today

One challenge we face is turning around public opinion to make aging research the number one priority. We need to overcome the denial about personal extinction that plagues the vast majority of the population. Once this is accomplished, I'm certain the collective efforts of the scientific community will deal with aging as efficiently as hand-held computers function today.

The other, more immediate challenge, is demonstrating the investment potential to wealthy individuals. Once we're able to demonstrate regeneration in animals and even return on early investments, both challenges should be easier.

We've designed two programs aimed at substantially increasing funding to entrepreneurs involved in age-reversal research.

But lack of believability may be our biggest roadblock. It's why revolutionary pursuits such as age-reversal don't happen on time. The solution is to educate those with the wherewithal to make them happen.

Remember the TV nature shows where a lion chases a huge heard of zebras, catches the slowest and then eats it? Did you ever wonder why the zebras don't simply band together, turn on the lion, and stomp it to death? Instead, they continue the bloody sacrifice, generation-after-generation, without ever thinking of chasing the lion away.

How programmed they are! How uncreative! How dumb! But are we any different?

Don't we stand around like dumb zebras watching 100,000 of our fellow human beings drop every day? We even wait meekly for our turn. Why aren't more people questioning this insanity? Why aren't more centimillionaires and billionaires figuring out, that money can indeed buy more time? Are we that much enslaved to our assumptions?

Don't you think the average billionaire would make a significant investment in research if he or she believed there were high odds of gaining an extra youthful decade or two, let alone open-ended vitality? Of course I'm sure some would give their last dime if full rejuvenation would be the payoff. But they are not doing it yet. This is one of the great tragedies of our time. It's our job to educate those who can make a difference while they're still here to find out.

As I said, I think the primary roadblock to raising the investment funds we need is the lack of belief (and understanding) that we can indeed solve aging in our lifetime. But first, we need to get ultra-wealthy people's attention.

We're hampered by the fact that they get inundated with investment proposals and donation requests. So they protect themselves with gatekeepers. And as consumers, they are tired of solicitations for overhyped products that promise to be the "next big breakthrough in anti-aging." No wonder they are skeptical. So when we try to get fifteen minutes to demonstrate how and why our researchers have true scientific answers to the extreme life extension challenges, not just supplements or drugs that may possibly buy them a just little more time, we run into barriers to getting appointments.

Tragically, billionaires and paupers alike suffer and die prematurely because the ones who can make a difference have not yet learned what real science and emerging technologies have to offer. It's our responsibility, not their fault, because we have not yet managed to overcome the barriers to reaching them... and with the right message.

But is it just a matter of education and persuasion/belief that keeps more of them figuring out that money can indeed buy more time?

No. Persuasion for sure, but more and more are now learning about these emerging technologies. So why aren't they leading the charge?

Fear!

You might not think so, but just like most of us, the ultra-wealthy care what other people think. A great number of them didn't care at first. They took big and sometimes unpopular risks while amassing their fortunes. Then something usually happens. They grow conservative. They start playing on big stages, and they care what their peers and the public think of them.

As philosopher Ciaran Healy points out, people fear little personal humiliations. They fear being embarrassed. They fear breaking from the herd, being proven wrong and having people laugh at them.

This is why humans, rich and poor alike, build their cages, why they shy away from risk and adventure, from daring conjectures that go way beyond anything previously imagined.

Pioneers don't toe the line. They have the little, simple courage to stand alone.

But the conscious or subconscious need for approval of our peers and the public often keeps most of us in our "safe" zones.

This is natural. It's a genetically programmed, subconscious protective response to something unexpected or new. Our reptilian brains, which evolved over millions of years, developed this way to avoid danger... to ensure survival. But now that we're not exposed to primitive dangers, this automatic response can work against us.

Ironically, this subconscious safety-seeking response causes those who can make a difference to risk premature death. But to recognize and to resist natural responses, to stand up and support radical life extension like Larry Page and Peter Thiel, the champions can avoid the permanent security of their tombs.

Health and Wealth

Ironically, early investors in these technologies may not only be the first beneficiaries of their life extending properties, they may also be able to multiply their wealth from the potential returns from their investments. How would you like to own a piece of the company or companies that develop age-reversing treatments or products? What would a cure for aging be worth?

Sure, we can wait until large funding sources finally catch up. Meanwhile though, over 100,000 lives get snuffed out every single day from aging. A five-year delay equates to 185 million more lost lives! Even minor delays will result in the suffering and death of millions. Scientists tell us they can start making an impact with only a few million more dollars per year, so we simply can't wait for nature to run its course. A delay could cost you or a loved one your life.

So I urge you to do four things:

1. Incorporate the seven simple steps into your life and gain 5–20 years—or more—from the steps you practice now. You will create a brighter tomorrow for yourself when you take some simple steps today.

2. Invest in some of these technologies. You can find current opportunities at www.MaxLife.org. Or you can donate to Maximum Life Foundation or SENS Research Foundation to support them. We have devised an offer that is so

irresistible that you may want to donate more than we can accept for that particular offer.

3. Keep abreast of advances and breakthroughs that could push you over the longevity finish line. Joining MaxLife keeps you ahead of the curve, so you can anticipate, prepare and take advantage of new developments. We'll send you regular updates at your request.

4. Above all, discover the Manhattan Beach Project. Just as the Manhattan Project put an abrupt end to World War II, The Manhattan Beach Project will let you age without aging. See what others are doing to turn this into a reality, see what you can do, and learn how you can benefit. Before landing on the moon, what did we do? We visualized it, imagined it and then dictated it. That's what MaxLife has now done for age reversal. Go to www.ManhattanBeachProject.com.

My worst nightmare is lying on my deathbed, knowing I could have done something to delay or avoid death, but didn't—or losing someone I love because I didn't try!

Remember those 100,000 people we lose prematurely to aging every day. When they vanish, so do their wisdom, experience, knowledge and skills.

I want you to be healthy, happy and prosperous, and I want you to live as long as you want. I want health and happiness for your family and loved ones, because Maximum Life Foundation believes we could demonstrate control over human aging and disease by 2033—pending funding. And that includes having the ability or being on the threshold to completely reverse aging damage. In other words, transforming your body into the shape you were in when you were in your twenties. Actually, better.

Of course, that's no guarantee, and it's certainly no reason to get complacent. The original projection was 2029, but the funding is not yet in place. (In those four extra years, 148 million more people will die from aging.) It could be thirty years… or forty… or even longer. Forty years or longer would surprise me, but it could take that long.

However between now and then, we will surely develop treatments and technologies that will expand your remaining lifespan.

That means medical science won't stand still in the interim. You'll continue to benefit from a breakthrough here, and a therapy there, and who knows? Before you know it, you may find yourself in a high-tech futuristic clinic undergoing full rejuvenation therapy.

This is literally "do or die." Dying is easy. Anyone can die. Living takes work. Living a radically long time takes even more work. We never had a choice before. It was always just a dream. But in our generation, the technology is catching up with this ages-old dream of extreme youth and longevity. Extreme healthy lifespans will be the norm someday. Staying alive long enough to benefit from these emerging technologies and to speed up their development takes the most work.

But you only have to do it once.

As I see it, limitless opportunities in our lifetimes will ultimately depend on several factors: (a) how much funding we can raise; (b) how soon we can raise the money; (c) how well you take care of yourself in the interim and (d) your ability to dodge accidents, other trauma or epidemics. Don't wait until it's too late, and then wish you would have spent a little time, money and effort for prevention.

Instead, plan on always enjoying the prime of life, endless vitality and a keen mind that never fades.

EPILOGUE

Y ou wake up to the sound of waves crashing on the rocks. It's a beautiful morning in Maui. (But aren't they all?) You bought your second home as a present to yourself on your 100th birthday... 25 years ago today.

Your family has gathered to celebrate this milestone with you. As usual, you're the first one up. It seems you've been an early riser ever since you had your DNA optimized. As a matter of fact, you are completely and safely rested on just three hours of sleep.

You've got a full day planned. First, you and your partner are going to take your daily pre-breakfast two-mile swim. Then breakfast with your family on your estate. The clan promised you a cruise around the island, so you'll all board the tram to Lanai at 8 AM. When the boat returns to the dock, it's off to lunch at your favorite waterfront restaurant. Finally, back home. Your great-great grandchildren are excited to get the surfing lesson you promised them last year.

The year 2014 doesn't seem that long ago. But decades have passed. That was the first time you read Smart, Strong and Sexy at 100?

At first, you thought the prospect of living an extended, youthful life was just hype to get you to read the book. But you were aging rapidly and couldn't ignore those nagging, telltale signs; arthritic knees and hips, lack of energy, anemic sex drive, wrinkled and sagging skin, hair loss—not a pretty picture.

You also recognized that accelerated progress was leading to new breakthroughs all the time... so, certainly there must be steps you might take to at least buy yourself more time. When you read it cover-to-cover, you took the super longevity predictions with a grain of salt, yet fortunately, adopted the seven life extending steps.

It wasn't long before you started looking and feeling better than you had in years. Even though you were not quite sold on the prospect of full age reversal, you couldn't help thinking of the possibilities. In fact, you even invested in the life sciences sector, targeting aging. Your result? The Maui estate and your financial independence.

Looking back, you remember the rejuvenating path you followed. Now it's hard to remember exactly how it felt to need reading glasses, the aches and pains you experienced as you aged and your fear of losing your independence during the downward spiral of growing old. But just in the nick of time, research yielded full age reversal.

You hung on years longer than you ever thought possible. In fact, even though you started slowing down, you swam and jogged into your 90's and never suffered from the serious health issues that took your parents and grandparents when they were much younger.

You recall facing those issues and symptoms at an early age and how you reversed the course with your lifestyle changes. Then, after you lived well past the ages when your parents and grandparents died, more and more legitimate anti-aging products came on the market, and your aging seemed to stop.

Now, at 125, you look better than you did when you were 35 and you feel and function better too... lots better.

The two big breakthroughs matured years ago, nanomedicine and genome reengineering. Even though regenerative medicine and tissue engineering, along with a wide variety of drugs and supplements, partially reversed your aging process, nanomedicine completely transformed you. They matured in time for you, thanks to MaxLife sponsored big artificial intelligence advances.

Now, thanks to nanotechnology and engineered improvements to your genome, you have more energy than you ever imagined, and you're much stronger, smarter and more durable than ever before. Time continues to march on, but you age without aging. You still marvel at your complete physical and mental restoration. Even after all these years, you haven't grown used to looking as young as your children and even your grandchildren. But you still take pride in your ability to put a smile on your partner's face more than a few times a week.

Of course, you cherish every moment. Your mind is sharp and your memory clear. You never get sick and never expect to.

Your investment in life science technologies has produced the ultimate ROI; a perpetual life enriched with youthful beauty, vitality and wealth beyond any you hoped for... or, even imagined.

Best of all, you have freedom. Your independence let you go back to school and to pursue your life's passion.

Now, you're stress-free and busier than ever. Your work is your play, and your play is your work. You enjoy a loving family and friendships that may never end. You found peace and happiness.

They used to say youth was wasted on the young... today, youth is for everyone.

Life is good.

LIVE LONG AND PROSPER

This part isn't about life extension at all, at least not directly. However, in my humble opinion, it's as important. In fact, the ideas you'll get here actually led me directly to my life's passion—life extension pursuits.

This has more to do with philosophy. When you master it, and when you finally manage to internalize all the lessons that follow, good health should be routine, both physical and mental.

We at Maximum Life Foundation look at life through holistic glasses. Longer life could be a curse without a clear sense of purpose, and a curse if you're not getting out of life what you should. More time magnifies destructive habits. This information will help delete any deficiencies, unhappiness, boredom and stress from your life.

But extra time also enhances all the good things you deserve and experience in life. That's why, since you plan on living for a very long time, it's even more important to master the life habits that contribute to your overall happiness and wellbeing. If you're like me, you'll need an extra hundred years to master them. Take them one at a time, and remember we're only human and will never reach perfection. But we can do our best.

This wrap-up points you in the direction of maximizing your happiness. It contains a summary of just about every meaningful thing I ever learned about life.

You'll profit from these nuggets.

More life!
David A. Kekich

P.S. MaxLife's philosophy can be summarized as "Enjoy today... and live one more day... for as long as possible."

KEKICH'S CREDO

1. People will do almost anything to stay in their comfort zones. If you want to accomplish anything, get out of your comfort zone. Strive to increase order and discipline in your life. Discipline usually means doing the opposite of what you feel like doing. The easy roads to discipline are: 1) setting deadlines, 2) discovering and doing what you do best and what's important and enjoyable to you and 3) focusing on habits by replacing your bad habits and thought patterns, one-by-one, over time, with good habits and thought patterns.

2. Cherish time, your most valuable resource. You can *never* make up the time you lose. It's the most important value for any productive happy individual and is the only limitation to all accomplishment. To waste time is to waste your life. The most important choices you'll ever make are how you use your time.

3. Think carefully before making any offers, commitments or promises, no matter how seemingly trivial. These are *all* contracts and must be honored. These also include self-resolutions.

4. Real regrets only come from not doing your best. All else is out of your control. You're measured by results only. Trade excuses and "trying" for results, and expect half-hearted results from half-hearted efforts. Do more than is expected of you. Life's easy when you live it the hard way—and hard if you try to live it the easy way.

5. Always show gratitude when earned, monetarily when possible.

6. Produce for wealth creation and accumulation. Invest profits for wealth preservation and growth. Produce more than you consume and save a minimum of 20% of all earnings. Pay yourself first.

7. You're successful when you like who and what you are. Success includes achievement—while choosing and directing your own activities. It means enjoying intimate relationships and loving what you do in life.

8. Learn from the giants.

9. A little caution avoids great regrets. Expect the best and prepare for the worst. Keep fully insured physically and materially and keep hedged emotionally. Insurance is not for sale when you need it.

10. Learn the other side's needs, offer as little information as possible, never underestimate your opposition, and never show weakness when negotiating.

11. Never enter into nor invest in a business without a solid, well-researched and well-thought-out written plan. Execute the plan with passion and precision. Plan and manage your life the same way.

12. Success comes quickly to those who develop great powers of intense sustained concentration. The first rule is to get involved by asking focused questions.

13. Protect your downside. The upside will take care of itself. Cut your losses short, and let your profits run. This takes tremendous discipline.

14. The primary purpose of business is to create and keep customers. Marketing and innovation produce results. All other business functions are costs. Prospecting and increasing the average value and frequency of sales are the bedrock of marketing and business.

15. If it's not proprietary, it won't work. Pay only on performance. Proprietary interest is one of the most powerful forces ever known. Whatever you reinforce or reward, you get more of.

16. Competence starts with guaranteeing your work.

17. Life operates in reverse action to entropy. Therefore the universe is hostile to life. Progress is a continued effort to swim against the stream.

18. Find out what works, and then do more of it. Focus first on doing the right things, and then on doing things right by mastering details. A few basic moves produce most results and income.

19. Use leverage with ideas (the ability to generalize is the key to intellectual leverage), work, money, time and people. To maximize profits, replicate yourself. Earning potentials become geometric rather than linear.

20. Rationalizations are generally convenient evasions of reality and are used as excuses for dishonest behavior, mistakes and/ or laziness.

21. Always have lofty explicit plans and visualize them intensely. Assume the attitude that if you don't accomplish your plans, you will literally die! This type of gun-to-your-head forced focus, survival pressure mindset, no matter how briefly used, stimulates your mind, forces you to use your time effectively, and illuminates new ways of getting things done.

22. The value of any service you have to offer diminishes rapidly once it's provided. Protect your compensation before performing.

23. Incalculable effort and hardship over countless generations evolved into the life, values and happiness we take for granted today. Every day should be a celebration of existence. You are a masterpiece of life and should feel and appreciate this all the way down to your bones. Aspire to create, achieve and

build onto the great value momentum taking place all around you.

24. Enthusiasm covers many deficiencies—and will make others want to associate with you.

25. Working for someone else gives you little chance to make a fortune. By owning your own business, you only have to be good to become wealthy.

26. Religiously nourish your body with proper nutrition, exercise, recreation, sleep and relaxation techniques.

27. The choice to exert integrated effort or to default to camouflaged laziness is the key choice that determines your character, competence and future. That critical choice must be made continually—throughout life. The most meaningful thing to live for is reaching your full potential.

28. Keep an active mind, and continue to grow intellectually. You either grow or regress. Nothing stands still.

29. Most accomplishment (and problem avoidance) is built on clear persuasive communication. That includes knowing each other's definitions, careful listening, thinking before talking, focused questioning and observing your feedback. Become a communications expert.

30. Power comes from stripping away appearances and seeing things as they really are. Socialism appeals to psychological and intellectual weaklings. Identify and replace all external authorities with internal strength and competence. Take full control of, and responsibility for, your conscious mind and every aspect of your life. Being incompetent or dependent in any part of your life or business opens you up to sloppiness, manipulation and irrationality.

31. If there is not a conscious struggle to be honest in difficult situations, you are probably being dishonest. Characters aren't really tested until things aren't going well or until the stakes are high.

32. Do not compromise if you are right. Hold your ground, show no fear, ask for what you want, and the opposition will usually agree.

33. If the situation is not right in the long term, walk away from it. Maintain a long-term outlook in all endeavors. Live like you don't have much time left—but plan as if you'll live for centuries.

34. Invest only after strict and complete due diligence. Don't allow yourself to be rushed. Make important decisions carefully, consider your gut feelings—then pull the trigger.

35. Stress kills. No matter how painful in the short-term, remove all chronically stressful situations, environments and people from your life.

36. Keep your overhead to a minimum. Rely more on brains, wit and talent—and less on money.

37. Business is the highest evolution of consciousness and morality. The essences of business are: honesty, effort, responsibility, integration, creativity, objectivity, long-range planning, intensity, effectiveness, discipline, thought and control. Business is life on all levels at all times.

38. That which is most satisfying is that which is earned. Anything received free of charge is seldom valued. You can't get something for (from) nothing. The price is too high.

39. By adhering to a strong honest philosophy, you will remain guiltless, blameless, independent, and maintain control over your life. Without a sound philosophy, your life will eventually crumble.

40. No dream is too big. It takes almost the same amount of time and energy to manage tiny projects or businesses as it does to manage massive ones—and the massive ones carry with them—proportional rewards.

41. There is no such thing as "just a little theft" or "just a little dishonesty."

42. Lead by example.

43. Take full responsibility for your actions or lack of action. He who errs must pay. This is an easy concept to grasp from the recipient's end.

44. An hour of effective, precise, hard, disciplined—and integrated—thinking can be worth a month of hard work. Thinking is the very essence of and the most difficult thing to do in business and in life. Empire builders spend hour after hour on mental work, while others party. If you're not consciously aware of putting forth the effort to exert self-guided, integrated thinking, if you don't act beyond your feelings and take the path of least resistance, then you give in to laziness, make bad decisions and no longer control your life.

45. Out-think, out-innovate and out-hustle the competition, and vividly visualize yourself as winning before entering into every deal or competitive situation. Maintain a blood-smelling, fighter pilot life-or-death attitude when any deal gets near to a close.

46. First impressions are lasting impressions. Put your best foot forward. People treat you like you teach them to treat you. A success key is positioning yourself at the top of their agenda.

47. The right thing is usually not the easy thing to do. You may sacrifice popularity for rightness, but you'll lose self-esteem for wrongness. Don't be afraid to say "no."

48. If someone lies to you once, he'll lie to you a thousand times. Lying is for thieves and cowards.

49. Have strict and total respect for other people's property.

50. Producing results is more important than proving you're right. To get things done, try to understand others' frames of references, points of view, needs and wants. Then determine what is honest, fair, effective and rational—and act accordingly.

51. Long-term success is built on credibility and on establishing enduring loving relationships with quality people based on

mutually earned trust. Cut all ties with dishonest, negative or lazy people, and associate with people who share your values. You become those with whom you associate.

52. Don't be preoccupied with things over which you have no control, and don't take things personally.

53. Spend more time working "on" your business than "in" your business.

54. Don't enter into a business relationship with anyone unknown to you without being furnished with references dating back at least ten years. If he or she doesn't have good enduring relationships, stay away. Check all representations on which you will rely made by everyone.

55. Enjoy life. Treat it as an adventure. Care passionately about the outcome, but keep it in perspective. Things are seldom as bleak as they seem when they are going wrong, or as good as they seem when they are going well. Lighten up. You'll live longer.

56. Identify exactly what it is you want. This takes a lot of thought. Then don't let anything stand in your way of getting it.

57. You can get any job done through the sheer force of will when combined with uncompromising integrity and competence. Strong leadership is the key.

58. You are responsible for exactly who, what and where you are in life. That will be just as true this time next year. Situations aren't important. How you react to them is. You have to play it where it lies.

59. The foundation of achievement is intense desire. The world's highest achievers have the highest levels of dissatisfaction. Those with the lowest levels are the failures. The best way to build desire is to make resolute *choices* for the future.

60. Integrate every aspect of your life (body, mind, spirit, relationships, business) and each within itself. Integrating means understanding and digesting a process—and seeing relationships

among seemingly unrelated phenomena. It's a sign of innovative genius.

61. Never be deceptive when trying to achieve a personal gain. Shortchanging others results in loss of self-esteem.

62. If your purpose of life is security, you will be a failure. Security is the lowest form of happiness.

63. Never enter into a contract unless all parties benefit. But no partnership is ever 50/50. There will always be inequities.

64. Review the basics of your profession at least once per year.

65. Bitterness, jealousy and anger empower your enemies and enslave you. Negative thinking results in the destruction of property. It is anti-property, therefore anti-capitalistic and anti-life. It also erodes your health. Put things behind you, learn your lessons, and get on with your life.

66. Most people spend 90% of their time on what they're *not* best at and what they don't like doing—and only 10% of their time on their best and most enjoyable ability. Geniuses delegate the 90%—and spend all their time on their "unique ability."

67. High self-esteem can only come from moral productivity and achievement.

68. There are an infinite number of new opportunities. Actively seek them out, and position yourself to recognize and take advantage of them.

69. There is no such thing as a good idea unless it is developed and utilized.

70. For maximum profits, identify and market universal needs, wants and trends. Creating desire, satisfying needs and wants, and replacing problems with creative innovations are the essence of profit generation.

71. To maximize opportunities, seek and master the complicated. The major solutions you find will be surprisingly simple, and the competition is minimal.

72. Always have options. Options are a primary source of power. Power also comes from stripping away appearances and seeing things as they really are.

73. Nothing wins more often than superior preparation. Genius is usually preparation.

74. Patience is profitable. Achievement comes from the sum of consistent small efforts, repeated daily.

75. Persistence is a sure path to success with quality activities. Never, ever, ever give up.

76. "I will do this" is the only attitude that works. "I'll try" or "I think" doesn't work.

77. Always work on increasing the size of the pie, rather than just your portion.

78. Rewards are rare without risks, but take only carefully calculated risks. Make sure the odds are on your side.

79. The "how" you get it (with integrity) is more important than the "what."

80. Be explicit and semantically precise in all communications, agreements and dealings. Summarize and write down important discussions—and make sure all sides agree. Putting agreements in writing avoids misunderstandings. Memories are fallible, and death is inevitable (so far).

81. The best way to get started is to get started. Life rewards action—not reaction. Wait for nothing. Attack life. Don't plan to death or ask for permission, but act now and apologize later.

82. Question everything. Don't believe it's true or right just because it's conventional. Strip all limits from your imagination on every deal and look for an unconventional creative opportunity in every mistake, crisis or problem. Be flexible, and be willing to turn on a dime when advantageous.

83. Have fun. The single key to a successful happy life is finding a vocation you enjoy—one that excites you the most.

84. Nobody gets old by surprise.

85. When it's a matter of producing or starving, people don't starve.

86. You get what you expect, not what you want. Fill your life with positive expectations. Demand the best. Attitude and desire contribute to 90% of your achievement. Anyone can learn the physical mechanics.

87. The surest way to accomplish your business plans is making service to others your primary plan. The key to success is adding value to others' lives.

88. The source of lasting happiness can never come from outside yourself through consuming values—but only from within yourself by creating values. Producing more than you consume is the only justification for existence.

89. Unattended problems will not go away, but will usually get worse. Anticipate and avoid problems—or meet them head on at the outset. Overcome fear by attacking it.

90. Find an excuse to laugh every chance you get, especially when you least feel like it.

91. When someone makes a big issue about his honesty or achievements, he is probably dishonest or a failure.

92. Put the magic power of compound interest to work with every available dollar.

93. The best investment you will ever make is your steady increase of knowledge. Invest in yourself. Thirty minutes of study per day eventually makes you an expert in any subject—but only if you apply that knowledge. Study alone is no substitute for experience. Education is always painfully slow.

94. For each important action you take, ask yourself if you would be embarrassed if it were published. It takes a lifetime of effort to build a good reputation but only a moment of stupidity to destroy it.

95. You are exactly what you believe and think about all day long. Constantly monitor your thoughts.

96. Skepticism is a key to rational thinking. Be especially skeptical of your own cherished beliefs. You might be wrong— and things change.

97. Anxiety is usually caused by lack of control, organization, preparation and action.

98. The first rule of sharpening your mind is to be an alert and sensitive observer. Observation is the genesis of all knowledge and progress—and is the first and last step of every thinking man's tool—the scientific method. Assume nothing. If it can't be observed, it's not true. Never act on blind faith. Whenever something sounds too good to be true, it almost always is. Refuse to be swayed by emotion when it conflicts with reason.

99. Experience is not what happens to you. It's what you do with what happens to you. It takes a wise person to learn from his or her own mistakes—and a genius to learn and profit from the mistakes and experiences of others.

100. The purpose of life is to delay, avoid and eventually *reverse* death.

Special Gratitude to:

Dr. Andrew J. Galambos	Gary C. Halbert	Joe Paterno
Dr. Wallace Ward	Sir Isaac Newton	Dr. Yul Brown
Frederick Mann	Michael Gerber	Patrick Malloy
Dr. Craig C. McGraw	Winston Churchill	Vince Lombardi
Daniel Sullivan	Napoleon Hill	Thomas J. Peters
George S. Clason	Bobby Jones	Harry Stottle

Anonymous (all those wonderful insightful heroes who influenced me one way or another, either consciously or unconsciously, but whose names I can't attach to any particular credo).

PLAN B

O ur ultimate plan at Maximum Life Foundation is to preserve human life. Yours, ours—everybody's. In keeping with that mission, we will continue to seek out all the latest ground-breaking research on each of the topics covered in this book, and provide that information to you in an easy-to-read format.

What if we don't succeed in time for you, though? Or what if you get whacked by an accident, another trauma or get blindsided by a deadly infectious disease?

Far from a sure thing, but scientifically sound enough to work, is a medical rescue protocol called cryonics. If you're not familiar with cryonics, research has shown that dying is not an event as once thought. Rather, it's a gradual process that starts after, not when, our hearts or brain waves stop. Our cells die gradually, over time. Cryonics is the methodology that halts this dying process with low-temperature technologies, stemming from the field of cryobiology. Contrary to popular belief, cryonics is simply an extension of modern medicine.

Remember when people were pronounced dead as soon as their hearts stopped beating? Physicians of the future will rarely pronounce people dead and will only do so after all advanced rescue technologies fail.

If the cryonics rescue team of today reaches patients in time after legal death, they may be able to place them into suspended animation, until such time as cures for what "killed" them are developed, and when age reversal technologies are mature. At that time, they plan on fixing you and waking you up.

A long-shot? Maybe. Wacky? If you think so, consider this:

Cryonics depends largely on two technologies. One is cryobiology, a well-proven field that deals with ultra-low temperatures. In this case, that means storing human tissue at liquid nitrogen temperatures for future therapies. This has been routine for many years.

The other is neurobiology, again, a totally legitimate and non-controversial field.

So it follows that it is just as legitimate to store and recover the brain (where your memory resides) while most of the cells are still alive as it is to store and recover any other tissue. So cryonics should work.

But your odds get even better.

Add another emerging, and soon to be maturing tool—regenerative medicine. We're already growing replacement organs, and soon, they promise to be as good as, or even better than the originals. You have read a little about regenerative medicine in Chapter Four during the stem cell discussion. Again, a well-accepted field.

As these technologies are fine-tuned, they may be more than enough for resuscitating patients. But there's more.

Another technology that may be enormously helpful for even more perfect rescue from suspension is nanotechnology. There's already more work in this field than I can ever hope to keep up with. Full-blown nanomedicine may be developed in as little as nineteen years. I mentioned nanomedicine in Chapter Four.

Finally, an ace in the hole is Artificial General Intelligence (AGI) as described in Chapter Four. If you read that carefully, you'll see the link between AGI and the ability to make something like cryonics work. Not only would it counteract most arguments against cryonics, but it should enable patients to be reanimated much sooner than almost anyone thinks possible. And don't forget the Law of Accelerating Returns. Don't you think having research tools a billion times more powerful in

25-30 years would make cryonics technologies enormously more viable, even without AGI?

Cryonics is not the extreme measure as some people mistakenly believe. It is actually the most conservative approach you can take if you are on the brink of death. Burial and cremation guarantee 100% cell death. Cryonics preserves your cells and gives you a chance to recover.

You need to plan ahead though, just like with traditional life insurance. In fact, you might look at cryonics preparation as the purest form of life insurance. Insurance is something you hope you never need but are glad you have when you do need it—when it's no longer for sale.

For more information, contact Alcor Life Extension Foundation at www.Alcor.org, or call 877-462-5267. They will send you a free information kit.

Smart, Strong and Sexy at 100? Should NOT Get Stale

Smart, Strong and Sexy at 100? is a continually evolving document. We make regular updates. The research on many fields mentioned here moves quickly, and we have plans to greatly expand the scope and detail of the material. When updates to this information are available, they can be found at www. MaxLifeSolution.com or on the Maximum Life Foundation website, www.MaxLife.org.

If there are topics you think should be covered in a future edition of this book, or if you have comments or questions about *Smart, Strong and Sexy at 100?* please feel free to contact us by going to www. MaxLife.org/sssbook and posting your comments. We are determined to find the best methods to keep you alive, young, and terrifically healthy until research programs halt and reverse the aging process.

How much value did you get from *Smart, Strong and Sexy at 100?* Who would you like to share it with? I encourage you to lend them your hard copy, refer them to www.MaxLife.org for a link to getting their own, or refer them to www.amazon.com or their local bookstore.

As more people digest this life extending information, more will benefit. Greater exposure also encourages donations to or investments in this research that can save your and their lives—and the lives of people you will never know. You will make a big difference by distributing as many copies as you can. You can also send them to www.MaxLifeSolution.com to register for a free copy.

Here's to your long, energetic, full, youthful and prosperous life!

–The Beginning–

APPENDIX A

How to Stop Your Aging Now

According to evolutionary biology authority, Dr. Michael R. Rose, before 5,000 to 10,000 years ago, mortality rates, or the rate of dying, increased steadily; in fact, exponentially, until around the age of fifty-five. Then they tended to plateau, and people's aging in some sense, stopped. The same thing happens to humans today, but we don't seem to plateau until around the age of ninety. This is where aging, or the progressive rate of mortality, levels out. But by then, our chance of dying in any given year is extremely high, even though some deterioration actually stops on its own.

We could thus keep people alive for a very long time after they plateau at around fifty-five. That means, their chances of dying at age eighty should be about the same as their chances were at fifty-five. The chances of us dying in any given year are low when we're in our 50's. Any serious health problems that might arise at that age should be infrequent, and we would be young and durable enough to survive medical interventions. Not so at age ninety and older. That's one reason hardly anyone ever lives to 110.

So if we could plateau in our fifties, sixties or seventies, we could be more active and live much healthier and much longer, in fact, *extremely* longer. The good news is we may be able to! In fact, in the new textbook, *Does Aging Stop?* by Laurence D. Mueller, Casandra L. Rauser and Michael R. Rose, these points are meticulously detailed with all the scientific rationale that aging can indeed stop, and our mortality rate can plateau! In fact, they hypothesize that not only can aging stop, but some aspects may decelerate as well. Although more research needs to be done, the evidence is convincing to me that if we can stop our accelerating mortality in our 50's, 60's or 70's, we may be able to live *indefinitely* with the help of modern medicine and its rapidly accelerating advancements.

Think about this implication:

One lifestyle change could allow you to live without limit within two years from the time you take action!

What are you waiting for? Here's the rationale behind this bold statement.

What happened 10,000 years ago? We entered the Agricultural Age. From 5,000 to 10,000 years ago, depending on your ancestry, we started growing crops and domesticating animals. That's when we started eating grains and legumes regularly plus dairy products, and we were not adapted to them.

We're far from completely adapted to agricultural diets now either, because 5,000 to 10,000 years is a short time on the human evolutionary scale. We are still adapted to the hunter-gatherer diet and active lifestyle. We've been on them for millions of years. We're also adapted to eating cooked meat and some cooked vegetables, since we've been eating them for well over a million years.

When we subsisted on a hunter-gatherer diet, we ate what we could find and kill. Those diets were actually much more diverse than typical modern diets. In fact, they may have been about *ten times* as diverse. While we typically select among about fifty different species today, our ancestors chose any of about five hundred! Because their selection was so varied, they tended to eat different foods every day.

In this variety of foods, a typical Paleolithic villager apparently ate on the order of 300 different plant species. Most modern diets include at most 30. We have a limited number of types of plant foods. In toxicology, the dose makes the poison, so the more you eat—if you eat a small amount of any toxin, your body will be able to eliminate it without any health effects. But if you eat a large amount, then it can become quite dangerous. When you eat any of the same food two days in a row or more, your immune system starts to recognize it as an invader. That's how your genes have evolved. So vary your food as much as possible.

Average hunter-gatherer life spans may have been short, mostly due to high infant mortality and partially due to the harshness and dangers of everyday life. But contrary to popular belief, *maximum* life spans may have been longer than the best we can hope to reach today if they could have enjoyed some of the security and medicine of the modern world. And diseases associated with aging were largely unknown.

Dr. Rose has hypothesized that by eliminating all grains, dairy products and legumes from your diet and by being physically active, you can reach your mortality rate plateau within two years if you are about fifty years of age or older. Then you could slow aging dramatically… drastically reduce your odds of falling victim to metabolic syndrome and be stricken with an aging-related disease. You could add an incredible number of healthy active years to your life, and even extend it open-endedly.

Even if he's wrong about plateauing (in order to be more objective, he used other scientists' plateau work to establish his hypothesis), in the worst case, this strategy will avoid more sickness and suffering than anything else I can think of.

According to *Does Aging Stop?* adaption is a function of age. We adapt well at early ages, but as adults age, we proceed back in evolutionary time. Sort of an evolutionary time travel. That means, you can tolerate, and even thrive, on an agricultural diet when you're young. But as you age, you become less tolerant to grains, dairy and legumes. If you're young now, there is no need to eat this way until you are over forty. In fact, it could be counter-productive for those much under thirty. But the older you are, the more damage an agricultural diet will do to you, and it may be deadly after age fifty if you don't reverse it.

The Human Diet's Three Overruling Principles

Based on the enormous information available to us, we can conclude that our original hunter-gatherer diet is based on three overruling principles:

1. It's exclusively whole food oriented.

2. It's primarily low glycemic.

3. It's inherently more vegetarian than carnivorous.

Although animal foods provide the highest quality protein, animal foods are not essential to us. Plant foods are. Vegetables, fruits, nuts, seeds and roots are our primary sources of vitamins and antioxidants. They're also exclusive sources of metabolic supportive phytonutrients.

Sure, a hunter-gatherer diet is not as convenient when you dine out. And it does take some trial and error and more creative grocery shopping. So the question you might ask yourself is, "Is it worth it?"

The answer is a no-brainer for me. "*Yes!*" Why? Because this diet is built into our genes. It is natural, and popular diets are not. Foods that agreed with hunter-gatherer genetic blueprints agree with ours. Eating a typical modern-day diet is like fueling a jet plane with diesel fuel. It will crash and burn.

There's an additional benefit too if weight loss is your goal. It's next to impossible to be overweight if you adopt a hunter-gatherer lifestyle for a protracted period of time. I noticed a marked increase in muscularity within sixty days. Others commented on it as well. Although I am already thin and do not want to lose weight, I have gotten noticeably leaner. The same thing happened to a female friend of mine who started the same time I did. However, if you are underweight, you may want to be cautious with anything that could cause weight loss.

I have another friend who reversed some serious health issues within seven months from the time he started a strict hunter-gatherer diet.

It works.

Another's Perspective

Steven B. Harris, M.D. looks even deeper into hunter-gatherer eating habits. His investigation shows that after mid-life (say 40), the evolutionary pressure is so small that EVERYBODY must switch to the Paleolithic diet and eat a hunter-gather diet like a Bantu (a lot of roots, fruits, and lean game-type meat or fish). If they don't, they get the kind of obesity that causes chronic disease (diabetes, cancer, vascular disease, etc).

It isn't that nature cares about what happens to you in this period (evolution is done with you), but rather that you do better sticking to the type of diet that didn't make you ill or fat in the reproductive years (age 15-35 or so) when it did matter evolutionarily. That's the tricky idea.

However, at ages over 40 where evolutionary pressure is small, our short species-experience with non-hunter-gatherer diets makes it very unlikely that we get anything out of agricultural diet. Instead, nearly all of us are stuck with having to go back to our Paleolithic roots, simply because the diet that doesn't make you too fat when young is also the one that doesn't do so when middle aged and elderly.

Since 1975, we've been in a food era which isn't Paleolithic or Neolithic but some monstrous THIRD period. It's not "lithic" (rock using) at all, but techno-factory. It is starch broken down to glucose than isomerized, so half of it is fructose, as though it was fruit sugar, then fed in massive quantities (more than you could get from fruit, and far cheaper). The rest of the starch and protein is used to feed feedlot cattle, which make so much cheap fat that when you eat them, you get diseases the Amish and Egyptians never saw.

This era has only been here to some extent since the 1960s and took off with a vengeance since the 1970s when feedlots and high fructose corn syrup began to dominate the Western diet. This is the era of "The Clown, the King and Colonel" as Anthony Bourdain terms them. And it's the "McDonald's and Burger King and KFC diet."

In the 40 years it's been here, evolution has NOT had time to adapt to this even a bit, and it causes reproductive problems and gestational diabetes even for people whose ancestors were farmers. This is the other tricky point. And moreover, for Native Americans and some segments of Africans, it's even worse! It's not safe or helpful at any age, but for some segments of the world and the gene pool, it's especially bad.

Here's How to Make It Work for You

I believe the following information is the single most important thing you can do for your longevity, bar none. If you take nothing else from this book, incorporate this step into your life.

As I said, for millions of years, we subsisted on a hunter-gatherer diet. That means we ate what we could find and kill.

By eliminating grains, dairy products and legumes from your diet and by being physically active, you position yourself to be able to avoid most of the aging-related diseases. Even if Dr. Rose's hypothesis about aging stopping proves to be wrong, you could still add lots of active years to your life by following this advice. You have everything to gain and nothing to lose. Find out more by reading *Food and Western Disease* by Staffan Lindeberg. This may be the single most important book you will ever read if your goal is extreme longevity. It's slightly academic, so I have synopsized some of the more pertinent points for you.

By studying how the human species evolved, Lindeberg and others developed a rational pathway to organize the conflicting ideas on the human diet. Their overwhelming evidence concluded that the Western diet is implicated in virtually every single chronic disease that afflicts us, and it specifically outlines the ultimate basis for the link between nutrition and disease.

All living organisms' nutritional requirements are genetically determined. By carefully examining the ancient environment under which our genome arose, it's possible to gain insight into which foods benefit us and which foods harm us.

The beneficial Paleolithic diet is mainly based on root vegetables, vegetables, fruits, berries, nuts, eggs, lean meat, poultry and fish. Paleo food contains a lot of water, fiber and protein which makes it filling at low calorie intake. A Mediterranean diet is a step, but only a step in the right direction.

The Kitavan islanders from New Guinea (one of the few remaining hunter-gatherer peoples) are current models of humans' original lifestyle. They have NO evidence of heart disease, stroke, dementia, diabetes, obesity (in spite of abundant food supplies), high blood pressure or acne. And they rarely exhibit modern lifestyle conditions such as cancer, arthritis, hip fractures, myopia and tooth decay despite there being plenty of subjects in their 80s and older. One-hundred-year-olds look and act like they're in their 60's and 70's.

Harmful foods that cause these diseases include modern staples such as grains, legumes, dairy, refined fats, meat from non-grass-fed animals, sugar and salt. These were not, or were rarely available to hunter-gatherers, from whom we have inherited our genes, but they now provide the bulk of calories in most countries.

In fact, the USDA reports that the top nine foods eaten by Americans are:

- Whole cow's milk
- 2 percent milk
- Processed American cheese
- White bread
- White flour
- White rolls
- Refined sugar
- Colas
- Commercial ground beef

All of these foods are foreign to our genome that evolved on a Paleolithic diet. This diet creates altered patterns of gene expression that lead to disease, including food allergy or sensitivity.

Grains and legumes destroy us in a number of ways. Plants contain toxic carbohydrate binding proteins called plant lectins that are designed to protect the plants against plant-eating animals.

They poison predators to discourage them from eating the plants. The highest concentrations are found in grains (except for cooked rice), beans, potatoes and peanuts. You'll find toxins in raw celery as well. Plant lectins are thought to be a major contributor to most modern diseases such as heart disease and cancer.

Since all plants contain lectins in varying concentrations, and since each contains its unique versions, you should eat a wide variety of fruits and vegetables in order to avoid concentrations of any one lectin high enough to harm you.

Our ancestors gravitated toward the plant foods that tasted best. Over time, we became more adapted to these foods and their defense mechanisms. This may be one reason we are not as adapted to raw celery as we are to blueberries. We're engineered to favor sweets. Companies like Coca-Cola, Kellogg's and Mars figured this out long ago.

Grains and beans also contain protease inhibitors which inhibit protein-degrading enzymes in the digestive tract.

Phytic acid is found in grains and beans as well. It binds to minerals and trace metals and passes them through the digestive tract and keeps them from being absorbed.

Dairy is about as destructive. Casein, the major protein in milk, and lactose, the largest constituent in milk by weight next to water, are proven to be major aggravators and producers of atherosclerosis. Milk contributes to diabetes in most ethnic groups and contributes heavily to arthritis and other inflammatory conditions.

Lactose intolerance is the natural genetic state for humans. Like all mammals we're genetically programmed to lose the ability to digest milk after childhood. It's part of the weaning process. Except for a few populations around the world who have independently developed genetic mutations that let them tolerate milk, most of us get undermined by dairy products.

Do you see some of the ways grains, legumes and dairy kill us? Yet they are staples of recommended diets in the Western world.

Today, it's natural to die of a heart attack, which was almost unheard of before the Age of Agriculture. "Normal" blood pressure means you are at "normal" risk for a heart attack or stroke. Blood pressure and body weight should *not* increase with age.

They only "normally" increase in sick populations. The majority of Westerners over sixty have *fully developed* atherosclerosis. So this again is "normal" for those of us with "normal" levels of blood pressure and serum lipids. Do you rejoice when your doctor says you are normal? The good news is, atherosclerosis is reversible in many cases by adopting a Paleo lifestyle.

If you have a health condition, gradually ease into a Paleo diet under the supervision of a *qualified and informed* physician.

Getting Started

Don't forget, if you're young now, there may be no need to eat this way. In fact, it could be counter-productive for children. But since adaptation drops drastically as we age, an agricultural diet after age fifty could cause your undoing. So if you're over forty, and especially fifty, start now if you want to optimize your health and longevity.

Most of the habits I describe in this book can be fairly easy to implement once you grasp the incredible benefits. In fact, they can even be fun, especially once you experience the results. I thought this one would take lots of willpower though, at least for me.

I used to enjoy a cup of chocolate ice cream every so often, and I do like cheese. But I have found good healthy alternatives. Even though they're not quite the same, I have discovered natural homemade non-dairy ice creams that almost make me forget traditional ones. Or if you want a commercial version that tastes like the real thing, try a coconut milk "ice cream." I was completely fooled by a product called So Delicious Dairy Free. And it only has one gram of sugar per serving.

Although I seldom touched bread, I thought it would be tough to figure out how to replace my oatmeal and whole grain cereals. Well, I was wrong. I even found grainless alternatives to both bread and cereals. For example, you can get ones made from sunflower seeds. See www.LydiasOrganics.com for some tasty and healthy substitutes. My favorites come from www.TwoMomsInTheRaw.com.

The web is full of recipes for grain-free breads, cereals, flours and pancakes made from almonds, coconuts and more as well as sources and recipes for non-dairy cheeses. And who needs dairy when you can enjoy delicious and nutritious almond milk, coconut milk or hemp milk? As far as breakfast goes, I've learned to love refreshing and healthy homemade protein shakes with hemp-seed or egg protein powder; almond, coconut or hemp milk, raw eggs; fruit; flax seeds and other goodies.

This is not a perfect science. We do know that eliminating grains, dairy and legumes will put you on the surest path we know of to an open-ended lifespan. The rest is fine-tuning and more study. Lots of Dr. Rose's information, including specific food advice, is posted on a free website. Please visit www.MissingHumanManual. com for a wealth of information.

A Paleolithic diet positions you and me better to take advantage of the emerging age reversal and repair technologies described in Part I of this book by extending our average lifespans now. In my opinion, this is the greatest life-extender of them all. And yummies like cacao and avocado, or plants like them, and some honey have probably been in our diet for millions of years, so we are not talking total self-denial.

According to Dr. Loren Cordain in his best selling user-friendly book, *The Paleo Diet*, there are seven keys to the diet.

1. Eat animal protein.

    a. Author's note: What if you are a vegetarian? You can eliminate the meat if you can get adequate protein from eggs or plant sources. As many as 30% of us can do well on a vegetarian diet. But most can't.

    b. Author's note: A common misconception of a Paleo diet is it leans heavily toward meats. The truth is, our ancestors found plant foods to be much more abundant and obtainable, so meats usually made up a relatively small portion of their diets. Popular neo-Paleo diets are not representative of true Paleo diets, since they contain much more meat than was available to our ancestors. I suggest you limit your portions of red meat, chicken, fish and eggs to three or four ounce servings. And try to avoid animal protein every other day on average.

2. Eat fewer carbohydrates than most modern diets, but eat good carbs from fruits and veggies.

3. Eat a large amount of fiber from non-starchy fruits and veggies.

4. Eat a moderate amount of fat with more monounsaturated and polyunsaturated fats than saturated fats, and nearly equal amounts of omega-3 and omega-6 fats.

5. Eat foods with a high potassium content and a low sodium content, and do not add salt to your food (Author's note: unless your sodium level is low).

6. Eat a diet with a net alkaline load.

7. Eat foods rich in plant phytochemicals, vitamins, minerals and antioxidants.

The Paleo diet can be roughly summarized as "any food that can be eaten without being processed." That means no grains, dairy and legumes. If total adherence takes too much fun out of your life, indulge once a week or more. Adhere as closely as you are comfortable with. Read this book for a fun and easy education, and enjoy life.

APPENDIX B

FAQs—COMMON MISCONCEPTIONS ABOUT EXTREME LIFE EXTENSION

Aging increases the possibility of sickness and disability, increases human suffering, and kills us if nothing else does. There is no objection to longevity that comes close to touching the present horror of aging—the more than 100,000 people who die each and every day. Yet there are a number of common objections to curing aging. Most of these are unfounded myths and easy to disprove.

Most objections can be dismissed when you make the benefits of retarding aging more concrete. Adding 20-30 years to the human lifespan, by a pill that mimics the effects of caloric restriction for example, would mean delaying cancer, heart disease, stroke, Alzheimer's, etc. When framed in that light, the concerns typically raised against life extension begin to sound less compelling, even ridiculous.

Would living with a lower risk of death from cancer, stroke or heart disease decrease our appreciation of living? If so, is that then a reason to promote smoking, obesity and sloth?

Is it desirable to increase the job prospects of today's younger adults by ensuring their parents' generation are afflicted with stroke or heart disease a decade or two earlier? Is increasing the risk of morbidity and mortality a fair and reasonable strategy for tackling societal problems like unemployment? No, of course not.

But much work needs to be done to persuade people to think rationally about these issues rather than be governed by their knee jerk reactions to such cases.

Here are some of the most commonly raised questions and concerns about a possible cure for aging followed by my responses.

1. Won't life extension increase population and tax our planet's resources?

Most people forget that we have a problem today, and prefer not to think about the tremendous costs of Alzheimer's disease or heart problems and the like. Instead, they express concerns about the kinds of hypothetical disadvantages envisaged for a post-aging world such as overcrowding.

Amazingly enough, when you factor out immigration, industrialized countries are actually seeing population declines rather than increases. However, even though our current resources and technologies could support 6 billion more people (according to world renowned economist Julian Simon), these concerns should still be addressed.

Life extensionists are generally responsible, problem-solving people who share these concerns. And the longer we keep them alive, the more brainpower we have to see these problems through, by developing better technologies for cheaper and more plentiful food and water, pure air, clean abundant energy and affordable housing.

Just as technology extends lives, it makes life more livable for larger populations. Since the Industrial Revolution, alarmists screamed doom and gloom about overcrowding and limited resources (backed by their "statistics"). However, the opposite has happened. The population increased by 740% since then, and standards of living have soared. It's not so much a question of resources as it is one of education, individual productivity and distribution—social problems, not life-extension problems. As long as people produce more than they consume, it's impossible to run out of resources.

In fact, Julian Simon also recognized that there is only ONE resource—Human Ingenuity!

Telling people they should die to make room for others is not a good solution to any problem.

2. Isn't it against God's will to tamper with nature?

What about antibiotics, organ transplants, laser surgery and all the other "miracles" we take for granted today? We heard these same arguments against such advances as anesthesiology for childbirth. To be human is to struggle against nature. If we were to follow nature's will, you probably wouldn't be here. Would God give us the ability to make life healthier and longer without wanting us to use it? Wouldn't God want to give us all the opportunity to choose life? Why would God create man with a mind able to enjoy so much and then frustrate him with a lifespan that allows him to experience so little? Wouldn't it be a sin to suppress life-giving technologies?

Finally, aging is not universal. A number of complex species such as lobsters, rockfishes, some tortoises and some plants do not appear to age. So aging is not a prerequisite to life.

Death is not the natural order of things. Overcoming death is.

Nature created the plague, polio, smallpox, cancer and more, but we don't see anyone suggesting we ignore these life shorteners.

For conscious intelligent beings, indefinite life eventually becomes the natural order.

3. Why would anyone want to live forever?

"Forever" is a long time, and we're not suggesting that. Most people who enjoy life want more of it. Even most of those who claim they don't want to live longer than "natural" will do anything to cure themselves of cancer, heart disease and injuries when they get stricken. Modern drugs, surgical techniques and diagnostic tools are life extension technologies that few refuse.

Most who welcome death suffer from the ravages of aging that usually make life miserable toward the end of their lives. We aim to avoid or reverse those side effects of aging. But as long as your life is fulfilling, now or in the future, why would you want it to end?

4. Wouldn't stopping aging simply extend my decrepit frail years?

Not at all. Our plans are keeping the young youthful and reversing the damage aging does to you if you are already affected by the ravages of aging. No one is interested in spending endless years in a nursing home. Age reversal will eventually mean transforming the elderly to a healthy youthful state. We aim to reset our biological clocks while our chronological clocks keep ticking.

5. Shouldn't we spend our resources feeding the hungry, rather than keeping people alive longer?

A knowledgeable human being is the ultimate resource. The elderly are the most knowledgeable people we have. By making them productive for extra years, many of those resources can be channeled to solving problems such as hunger. Besides, our planet can accommodate over 12 billion people before resources are taxed. This doesn't even account for future technologies such as seabed farming, mining asteroids, clean energy-saving technologies, mile high buildings (Frank Lloyd Wright designed one in 1956 that could have housed all of downtown Chicago. Imagine the views!), enhanced food production, nanotechnology and genome engineering.

What's more, the exponential progression of information technology as explained in Chapter Two will affect our prosperity as well. The World Bank has reported, for example, that poverty in Asia has been cut in half over the past decade due to information technologies, and that at current rates, it will be cut by another 90% over the next decade. That phenomenon will spread around the globe.

Finally, you can use this irrational argument against any expense or investment. Should we divert resources from developing cancer drugs or cleaning the environment, to feeding the hungry?

6. How can you expect to solve something as complex as aging, when we can't even cure cancer?

For a couple of reasons. First, it may not be necessary to solve something as complex as aging in the near future. Fixing the damage aging causes may not be nearly as complex. That may be all we have to do to build a "bridge" between today and the day we can enjoy the benefits of technologies that control the aging process.

Second, we already have some pretty compelling clues as to what causes aging—enough in fact, to put our version of a biological "Manhattan Project" to work right now. We even know how to extend average lifespans by up to twenty years in many people using current low-tech lifestyle modifications. Unraveling the aging mystery was an unrealistic project just a few years ago, but recent giant technological and computational leaps give us the tools to make it a reality. For example, some biological problems used to take years to solve. Now they take about fifteen seconds. These tools will only get better faster with exponential growth of knowledge and technology.

Then don't forget, some organisms such as the **hydra** show no evidence of aging at all. And planarian flatworms appear to exhibit an ability to live indefinitely.

7. Won't longer lifespans threaten the Social Security system, Medicare and pension plans?

Yes, as they're structured today. But remember, average lifespans have increased steadily and dramatically most of this century. In fact, U.S. average lifespans increased by twenty-nine years since 1900. Governments and industry successfully adjusted to it. The greatest burden on healthcare comes from the elderly. If aging is not tackled, societies will consist of a large portion of frail, elderly people, which will result in a serious financial burden. Our mission is to avoid having elderly patients and to keep them youthful and productive. So curing aging would be economically sound. People would live longer but also work longer and be more productive. Without the declining years of old age, healthcare and the economy would benefit from a cure for aging.

Sure, change sometimes hurts, but aren't millions of premature deaths a high price to pay to keep retirement and entitlement plans static? Besides, shouldn't each individual be offered that choice for his or her life? Wouldn't it be immoral to suppress or withhold life extending technology, because some people want to protect the status quo?

8. What will we do with all the "old people"?

"Old people" can be our most valuable resources. We generally acquire more experience, knowledge, wisdom and skills as we age. Rather than putting us "out to pasture" or in nursing homes, wouldn't society be better off if we kept ourselves youthful and productive? On average, people spend more on medical bills during the last year of their lives than all the rest of their years combined.

9. You don't need modern technology. Won't meditation, yoga, exercise, supplements, faith and pure food, air and water accomplish the same thing?

Only to a degree. These can all help us live longer, but no one has ever been proven to live beyond 122 years. We plan to extend the maximum lifespan, while allowing people to be active and youthful well into "old" age. In the meantime, keep up your healthy habits.

10. Why hasn't the medical community gotten behind a treatment for "aging" by now?

Mainly because the vast majority of people don't see aging as a disease, let alone a solvable one. Imagine the urgency that goes into freeing victims trapped beneath a collapsed building. Aging is equally disastrous, but on a scale magnified by a factor of millions. Yet, because it sneaks up on us, and because hardly anyone recognizes aging as treatable, most people accept "natural" death—and die.

11. Won't only the rich be able to afford extreme life extension technologies?

Maybe. But if so, only at first. Today, we experience about a 50% annual deflation factor for many if not most technologies. And this factor keeps increasing. In other words, technologies get more affordable faster, at an ever-increasing rate. Only the wealthy can afford many new technologies. But at that stage, they usually don't work very well. At the next stage, they are affordable to many people and work better. Soon, they work well and are affordable to most. Finally, they're almost free. The progression from mostly unaffordable technologies to very inexpensive is currently about ten years. Ten years from now, it will be about five years. And twenty years down the road it will only be about a two to three year lag.

12. Won't life be boring if we live a long time?

If you're bored now, maybe. But as we advance in every area of life, we see more and more opportunities and more and more diversity. This is continuing, not decreasing. Imagine the opportunity to spend active time with your children's great, great grandchildren. How about embarking on a new career or going back to school and studying something you really love? I believe bored people have either lost hope or they are doing something outside of their passion. If you had an open-ended future to pursue your dreams, would you be bored? Also consider the prospect of enhanced intelligence. Without it, maybe living for hundreds of years or longer would get boring. And virtual reality will open up whole new worlds and experiences to you. You will surely enjoy extreme life expansion along with extreme life extension.

13. I wouldn't want to outlive all my friends.

Consider this likely scenario: *You* may be the one left behind, while your friends and family stay together long into the future. Also, this phrase, at least to me, is an illogical reason for a death wish. First, if we have a choice, and your friends choose to die, why would you let them drag you along? Second, if you're like me, you continually meet new people. Many become friends. And a few become close friends. How many new friends do you think you could make in several more lifetimes? How many people do you know who lost close friends or family members or who went through emotionally draining divorces and still found happiness and even new and better relationships? Heartbreak and loss eventually heal, and there are lots of interesting people in this world who would love to know you.

Simply put: Life is Good, and Death is Bad.

APPENDIX C

THOUGHTS AND QUOTES FROM SCIENTISTS AND LIFE ENTHUSIASTS

"With quite modest resources, we should be able to control and reverse aging in mice within a decade. I predict that once this has been done, humanity will no longer need persuading to work as hard as possible to translate that success to humans. Thus, substantially extending mouse lifespan with late-onset interventions is my key medium-term goal. The Methuselah Mouse Prize, and especially the Reversal Prize, is a powerful way to make that happen sooner."
—Aubrey de Grey

"In life, we face many challenges. Solving or avoiding the obvious problems, leads us to the ultimate problem. Aging is the ultimate problem.

"Such research is critical if developed countries are to avoid the financial crisis now threatening as the baby boom generation reaches sixty-five and begins the decline in health that causes 90% of their lifetime medical expenses to occur during the last 10% of their lifespan. The huge financial and social dimensions of this problem dwarf those of social security, and could cause inflation and bitter divisions as the aged compete for drugs, artificial limbs and organs, heart pumps and other devices that will be developed as progress continues in pharmaceuticals, biotech and bioengineering."
—Paul Glenn

"I believe we are biologically designed to hate death and fight it. What makes us different from other creatures we're aware of is that we can anticipate that a future will come to be.

"Every single human being on the planet—including my children—will experience the disaster of involuntary aging—unless action is taken—today—by me. This will not be accomplished while I wait for 'someone else' to pay the bill.

"I can leave my children an inheritance of money or life. Which will you choose?"

—David Gobel

"There is nothing in biology yet found that indicates the inevitability of death. This suggests to me that it is not at all inevitable and that it is only a matter of time before biologists discover what it is that is causing us the trouble and that this terrible universal disease or temporariness of the human's body will be cured."

—Richard Feynman, Nobel laureate

"I am a funeral director by trade and have seen more than my share of death. It is never pretty, and some of the things I have seen are terrifying. If you have ever thought about how peaceful someone looked in a casket, let me let you in on a little secret, they didn't look that way before we embalmed them. I have yet to pick someone up from the morgue that looked glad to be there.

"The day will come for most of us when death approaches and we will go through a list of things we wish we had done. If only I had started my diet earlier, why didn't I keep my New Year's resolution to exercise?

"Before you know it, one of my friends or I will be coming for you. Put us out of work before we do."

—David Thompson

"[Aging] takes healthy vigorous people who can take care of themselves, and it turns them into frail weaklings who require lots of (expensive) supportive care until they expire from some condition to which it has made them more susceptible. I've been spending a lot of time in nursing homes lately, and it's quite obvious that the people there have something wrong with them; to suggest otherwise is, I think, little more than a species of denial. Aging is a disease, a disorder, a killer. We should be doing something about it."

—Glenn Reynolds

"We are at a societal tipping point similar to the one that occurred for cancer research in the late 1960s and early 1970s. Slowly, the public is beginning to realize the possibilities offered by future medicine.

"Through education, awareness and high-profile sponsorship of science, we can bring about widespread support for real anti-aging research and the funding to make it happen.

"The future of individual health and longevity is in our hands. It is our voices and our dollars that ultimately determine whether therapies are researched, whether cures are developed. If we don't raise our voices, then the future will be shorter and less healthy for each and every one of us."

—Reason, Founder, Longevity Meme

"The planet is in the grip of a killer disease that is invisible to most, precisely because it is universal. Its name is *aging*.

"The toll in disability, suffering, dollars, and deaths attributable to the biological aging process is so enormous that the mind simply cannot take in the numbers. We need research designed to directly take on aging *itself*, rather than piecemeal attacks on individual age-related diseases, which yield ever-diminishing returns. But the science needed to push forward genuine anti-aging medical interventions is not being done, because of perverse structural defects in the way that biomedical research is funded. Venture capital's timescales are too short to see genuine anti-aging drugs through the development pipeline. And government-funded research bureaucracies are stuck in a political logjam, feeding and feeding upon the public's failure to make medical research into aging a political priority."

—Michael Rae

"Every day, my mailbox is filled with solicitations from worthy charities seeking contributions to cure a specific disease. While I applaud the efforts of these groups, I seldom contribute because the benefits seem to be conferred on such a narrow group of beneficiaries. Such charities by their nature tend to consume a large portion of their donations on further fundraising.

"My vision of an ideal charity aimed at health and longevity is one that seeks to do basic research about the causes and prevention of aging. This kind of basic scientific research seems to me more likely to produce the kind of dramatic breakthrough that will conquer all sorts of diseases and benefit the most number of people. These kinds of advances inspire me in their potential to foment a conceptual revolution about how we think about aging, disease, longevity, and life itself.

"Long life is the greatest blessing, but a long, healthy life is a greater blessing still. My first child, Timothy, arrived just a few days ago, and I want to spend many, many years with him."
—Mike McCormack

"The aging process is like the weather, only worse. Everyone complains about it, almost no one does anything about it, and very few people even try to do anything about it. Like many behavior patterns that were formed in our evolutionary past, this is irrational and inappropriate to our modern situation as an intelligent species.

"The process of aging and dying has robbed me of some of my dearest friends and has destroyed their infinitely precious skills, memories, knowledge and human values. The aging process is now busily destroying my own mind and body.

"Whatever social problems might be caused by a greatly increased lifespan, the benefits would be infinitely greater; and more to the point, for anyone who cares about human life, [intervening in] the aging process is our highest ethical obligation."
—Charles Platt

"Although fascination with the seemingly inevitable process of aging and with the attempts to postpone it is certainly not new, research in this area became particularly exciting during the last decade. Reports that mutation of a single gene can greatly extend lifespan in organisms ranging from yeast to mice raised a very real hope of discovering the fundamental processes that control aging and determine longevity. Particularly exciting is the possibility that this understanding may allow devising methods that would delay human aging.

"We are working with mutant mice in which reduced release of several hormones from the pituitary or resistance to the actions of one of these hormones are associated with very impressive (approximately 50%) increase in life expectancy. These animals not only live long but are also partially protected from cancer and other age-related diseases and maintain their memory and learning ability into very late life."

—Andrzej Bartke

"I'm already doing all I can to slow my own aging processes through Calorie Restriction, the only known way to slow aging in humans. But I'm not satisfied with holding back the inevitable, so I'm going to put my time, talent and resources into the search for the real solution.

"I'm not a scientist—I'm an organizer. I see the world as a series of relationships, in which we are all connected to and dependent on each other. I believe that what each individual does matters. If there's anything I can do to give just one more day of life and health to the people I love, I'm going to do it."

—April Smith

"Today, hardly anybody would settle for a lifespan of forty years (which was the average only some decades ago). Our current life expectancy of approximately seventy-five years will be equally unacceptable a few decades from now.

"In our complex and rich world, we only start to become productive close to age thirty and begin to feel the decline shortly thereafter. Let's expand this short time, go to all the places we ever wanted, learn all the hobbies, languages and friends that are out there!"

—Patrick Burgermeister

"One day the questions will be asked, 'Could we not have made this happen sooner?' and 'Why did hundreds of millions of people have to die prematurely?'

"Personally, I do not want to be among those who did nothing. I want to be among those who shared the vision and who cared enough to contribute to its realization. And if it happens in our lifetime, how wonderful that would be!"

—Nick Bostrom

"My mother died before she ever had a chance to meet her grandchildren. My father died when my son was one. When I look in my children's eyes I want to know them when they are old and wise, and I want to see what their children and their grandchildren accomplish. Some people think that the struggle for radical life extension is a selfish one, but I see it just the opposite. My political mentor, Michael Harrington, said that being a fighter for social justice was 'long distance running.' Michael died in 1989, before he could see the fall of the Berlin Wall, something he had longed for his entire life. Like Michael, I want not only to live more life myself, but to see what becomes of this world and do what I can to build a better one."

—James Hughes

"As far as I can tell, human beings won't be able to stop themselves from living longer. Whether it's for science or space travel, intelligence expansion or love, humans will express life's ultimate and most primal drive, to keep living."

—Devon White

"To the man of Reason, no knowledge of the universe is inherently beyond his grasp. Anything can be fathomed, formulated, analyzed, and explained by a mind with the training and the will to do so. But the mind must be present first. In death, the mind is destroyed, and, thus, the state of death is the only truly *unknowable* condition there is; no man can know what it is like to be dead. The *unknown* does not scare the Rational Man; he pursues it with the vigor of a conquering hero. But the *unknowable* must horrify him, for he is

left as its pawn and sacrificial fodder, and is ultimately destroyed by it. Let us not allow any more rational men to enter the state of death, of the unknowable, but rather attempt to thwart it while they still live and have a full ability to grasp the world before them. Let knowledge overcome annihilation!"
    —Stolyarov II

"Just walk into any nursing home and you see the tragedy unfolding."
    —Robert Wilkes

"I believe that everyone should have the choice to live longer. For those who live their lives to the fullest, the current average lifetime does not seem long enough to experience everything that life has to offer. I believe that what is needed is a concerted effort by the people who want to live longer to pursue this goal and also a dialogue with the people who fear living longer. For me, dying would be a waste of knowledge and life, but I do not fear it. It puzzles me why some people fear living longer."
    —John Cumbers

"This project arouses every primal instinct in me. Being alive is the ultimate aphrodisiac. It's sexy. And though there is a choir of good reasons to support this project, one comes most strongly to mind: *I love being alive.*
    "There are a lot of things that I want to accomplish in my life and might not be able to if aging gets to me first. I would hope that every little bit helps and maybe one day something can be done to prevent the effects of aging and prolong life. I am only nineteen years old, and I don't want to live forever, but a few extra years would be nice. It's a big world and there is a lot to see and learn."
    —Tanya Forcade

RESOURCES

Websites:

Alcor Life Extension Foundation is the world leader in cryonics, cryonics research, and cryonics technology. www.alcor.org

American Aging Association (AGE) promotes biomedical aging studies directed towards increasing the functional lifespan of humans. This site is geared towards health professionals. www.americanaging.org

Ben Best assembled an in-depth study of aging and how to overcome it since 1990. You'll find it all here. www.benbest.com

Better Humans offers a forum for life extension bloggers as well as a great collection of articles and videos. www.betterhumans.org

The Calorie Restriction Society helps people of all ages live longer and healthier lives simply by eating fewer calories and by maintaining adequate nutrition. www.crsociety.org

The Cryonics Institute is the second biggest company that offers cryopreservation services and information. www.cryonics.org

Does Aging Stop? See 55 bite-sized lessons on how a Paleolithic can halt aging. www.55theses.org.

Extropy Institute is a think tank ideas market for the future of social change brought about by consequential technologies. www.extropy.org

Fight Aging is one of the best and most complete resources you will ever find for practical, general, and scientific information on life extension. www.fightaging.org

Grow Young Guide emphasizes the joy in youthful living. www.howtogrowyounger.com

International Anti-Aging Systems is a leading international supplier of anti-aging products and information. www.antiaging-systems.com

H+ Magazine brings you the world's most exciting tech and futuristic information. Fun and easy to read. www.hplusmagazine.com

Dr. Joe Mercola's site shows you why an active, healthy lifestyle is easier than you think. It spells out how you can Take Control of Your Health! This is one of the most popular informative health and well-being sites on the Web. www.mercola.com

Life Enhancement Products is an innovative manufacturer of nutritional supplements with unique formulations. They have been avid supporters of extreme longevity since 1985. www.life-enhancement.com

Life Extension is a global authority on health, wellness and nutrition as well as a provider of scientific information on anti-aging therapies. They supply only the highest quality nutritional supplements, including minerals, herbs, hormones and vitamins. www.lef.org/maxlife

LifeStar Institute is dedicated to averting the pending global aging crisis in the pursuit of personnel, sciences and processes to develop therapies that restore knowledge and productivity. www. lifestarinstitute.org

Longecity takes the strongest stand on life extension to the extreme. You'll find a wealth of practical, current and futuristic information here. www.longecity.org

Maximum Life Foundation. That's us. www.MaxLife.org

MaxLife Solution supports companies and technologies designed to dramatically intervene in the aging process. MaxLife Solution sources a handful of the most powerful longevity supplements. www.MaxLifeSolution.com

The Methuselah Foundation formulated a group of detailed research proposals for repairing all known forms of aging-related damage to the human body. www.methuselahfoundation.org

Project LIFE aims to raise funding for a fast-track, large-scale, global, multi-disciplinary R&D effort focused on finding effective treatments to control aging within the lifetime of the funds contributors. www.projectlife.org

Ray & Terry's Longevity Program, described in their books, *Transcend* and *Fantastic Voyage: Live Long Enough to Live Forever,* counteracts the long standing imbalances in metabolic processes that are the leading causes of death. www.rayandterry.com

SENS Research Foundation works to develop, promote and ensure widespread access to rejuvenation biotechnologies which comprehensively address the disabilities and diseases of aging. www.sens.org

Vitamin Research Products opened in 1979, partnering in your health. They are a first class educational source with outstanding products. www.vrp.com

Recommended Reading:

100 Plus: How the Coming Age of Longevity Will Change Everything, From Careers and Relationships to Family and Faith by Sonia Arrison

Abundance: The Future Is Better Than You Think by Peter H. Diamandis and Steven Kotler

The Age of Spiritual Machines: When Computers Exceed Human Intelligence by Ray Kurzweil

The Biology of Belief: Unleashing the Power of Consciousness, Matter, & Miracles by Dr. Bruce H. Lipton

Body for Life: 12 Weeks to Mental and Physical Strength by Bill Phillips and Michael D'Orso

Countdown to Immortality by FM-2030, Flora Schnall and Dr. Aubrey de Grey

Ending Aging: The Rejuvenation Breakthroughs That Could Reverse Human Aging in Our Lifetime by Dr. Aubrey de Grey and Michael Rae

Engines of Creation: The Coming Era of Nanotechnology by Dr. K. Eric Drexler

Everyday Paleo: Embracing a Natural Diet & Lifestyle to Increase Your Family's Health, Fitness and Longevity by Sarah Fragoso

Fantastic Voyage: Live Long Enough to Live Forever by Ray Kurzweil and Dr. Terry Grossman

Food and Western Disease: Health and Nutrition from an Evolutionary Perspective by Staffan Lindeberg

The Future of Aging: Pathways to Human Life Extension by Michael D. West, L. Steven Coles, Stephen B. Harris, and Gregory M. Fahy

Green Smoothie Revolution: The Radical Leap Towards Natural Health by Victoria Boutenko

How to Create a Mind: The Secret of Human Thought Revealed by Ray Kurzweil

The Immortality Edge: Realize the Secrets of Your Telomeres for a Longer, Healthier Life by Greta Blackburn, Michael Fossel, M.D., Ph.D. and David Woynarowski, M.D.

The Life Extension Revolution: The New Science of Growing Older Without Aging by Dr. Monica Reinagel and Philip Lee Miller, M.D.

The Longevity Diet: Discover Calorie Restriction—the Only Proven Way to Slow the Aging Process and Maintain Peak Vitality by Brian M. Delaney and Lisa Walford

The Metabolic Plan: Stay Younger Longer by Dr. Stephen Cherniske

The Paleo Diet: Lose Weight and Get Healthy by Eating the Food You Were Designed to Eat by Loren Cordain

Ready, Set, GO!: Synergy Fitness for Time-Crunched Adults by Phil Campbell

Redesigning Humans: Our Inevitable Genetic Future by Dr. Gregory Stock

The Relaxation & Stress Reduction Workbook by Dr. Martha Davis, Elizabeth Robbins Eshelman, Dr. Matthew McKay, and Patrick Fanning

The Singularity Is Near: When Humans Transcend Biology by Ray Kurzweil

The Six Pillars of Self-Esteem by Dr. Nathaniel Branden

Strength for Life: The Fitness Plan for the Rest of Your Life by Shawn Phillips

Superfoods: The Food and Medicine of the Future by David Wolfe

Take Control of Your Health by Dr. Joseph Mercola and Dr. Kendra Pearsall

Transcend: Nine Steps to Living Well Forever by Ray Kurzweil and Dr. Terry Grossman

Younger Next Year: Live Strong, Fit, and Sexy - Until You're 80 and Beyond by Chris Crowley and Henry S. Lodge